THE HIDDEN DANGERS OF SOY

Dianne Gregg

Outskirts Press, Inc.
Denver, Colorado

DISCLAIMER

The Hidden Dangers of Soy is intended solely for informational and educational purposes and not as personal medical advice. Please consult your health care professional if you have any questions about your health.

DEDICATION

This book is dedicated my loving husband, Donald, for editing, assistance with research and footnotes, and having patience with me – even when he was carrying a full load of working two jobs and completing his studies for a PhD in Education for himself!

TABLE OF CONTENTS

ACKNOWLEDGMENTS

I would like to thank the following people for their support because without them, this book could not be accomplished.

Dr. Michael J. Duckett, my mentor, www.upgradinglife.com, for his continued inspiration, encouragement, advice, and support even when I felt overwhelmed.

Richard and Valerie James, www.soyonlineservice.co.nz, for their tremendous amount of input to enhance the research, and all the testimonials they provided me about others suffering from consuming soy products, especially infants consuming soy formula. I am truly grateful.

Kaayla T. Daniel, PhD, CCN, author of *The Whole Soy Story: the Dark Side of America's Favorite Health Food*, www.wholesoystory.com, for taking the time out from her busy schedule to review and note comments and corrections to my book where needed. I appreciate all your assistance.

And finally, yet importantly, my family, friends, and colleagues who supported me for having the guts to write this book.

INTRODUCTION

I have two main things I want to do in writing this book. The first is to share my personal experiences with you about how soy nearly killed me and how my soy-free life has improved. The second is to raise questions about the growing use of soy in just about every food product on our shelves today. I want to be fair to both sides of the soy question, but I don't feel I have to give a balanced account. I *want* to raise these questions. Your health and the health of your children depend on the answers.

I've researched this subject as a concerned citizen, and you will see that I have included research studies where they seem to be helpful. It's tough because so many studies are conflicting. I'll try to explain these studies, and I'll include references that will let you find the research and decide for yourself.

But I *am* on a mission. I want to help others maintain good health. There are many testimonials in this book from people who developed serious problems, and they sure don't think soy is a "health food"! I believe it is time for like-minded consumers to band together so we can make real changes in the food manufacturing industry.

As you read my story, you'll see how weight gain fits

into it. Women have been obsessed with their weight for years. They try one fad diet after another to lose weight. Unfortunately, they gain back the weight plus some. When we reach our mid-forties, it seems as though we start gaining weight, retaining water, and feeling bloated most of the time. Doctors tell us it's menopause, and we half-heartily accept it. Maybe you are developing a thyroid problem.

When you read my story and the research that went into creating this book, you'll be amazed at what you will learn. That's why this book isn't just for women – it's for everyone. I believe that all women will gain a lot from it, but some of the strongest warnings are for pregnant women and for mothers with infants and young children.

If you feel I've raised enough serious questions in the book, consider starting to make a difference. At the end of the book, I'll give you some ideas of how we can raise our voices and be heard. If you no longer want to buy some of the products I talk about and enough of us let the manufacturers know it, they will change their products back to what they were before the soy industry spent billions to convince them to use soy in their products. If there is no market for it, there is no point in putting soy in everything. We can change the world through our action, not by just talking about it.

ENDORSEMENTS

Would you knowingly eat something that causes nausea, gas pains and indigestion? That leads to hormonal imbalance, thyroid problems, gout and even cancer? That contains "bad" fats and other unhealthy substances? Something that has no positive effect on your heart whatsoever?

I certainly wouldn't. And neither should you. For years now, you've been hearing about the "miraculous" benefits of soy-based products. But the reality is far different: In its raw, unfermented form, soy is inedible and foreign to your body. It's not part of your native diet and your body has no way of successfully coping with it.

Dianne Gregg's book does a great job of clearly illustrating the dangers of soy and how the media has misinformed millions into thinking they're doing themselves a favor by consuming more and more soy products. This book is a much-needed wake up call and a must read for every American.

Al Sears, MD
Director, Center for Health and Wellness,
Wellington, FL
Author of *The Doctor's Heart Cure* and *PACE:*
Rediscover Your Native Fitness

As a Scientist and Physician with an extensive background in nutrition, I was feeding my children soy products. After being educated on the Dangers of Soy by Dianne Gregg, all soy products are out of the house--for good! Thank you so much for the powerful insight and valuable information you provide to the public. My children's allergies are greatly improved and we owe it to you, Dianne.

Dr. Michael J. Duckett
Upgrading Life.com

Dear Dianne, Thank you for your thoughtful advice about my health and treatment. I want to fight this fight with every resource available so I take all of your suggestions to heart as I chart my course. Your support means so much to me and to my family in keeping all of our spirits up. Thank you for all of your prayers and wishes.

Elizabeth Edwards

I found Dianne's approach in her book... "**The Hidden Dangers of Soy**" alternating between her "personal story" and her enumeration of the medical studies about soy products to be at once compelling as well as informative. Having completed a Nutrition Fellowship at Memorial-Sloan Kettering Cancer Center (as well as doing nutrition research at MIT as an undergraduate), I was impressed with her enumeration of the scientific data on soy products as thorough all the while maintaining a high degree of objectivity.

Leonard J. Weiss, M.D.
Board-Certified in Internal Medicine,
Psychiatry, Addictionology, Forensics,
and Nutrition.

Thanks to Dianne, I've lost 18 pounds in the past three months just by removing soy products from my diet. Now, when I go to the grocery store, I read the ingredients on the labels. If I see soybean oil, vegetable oil, etc...I put it back on the shelf and look for something else. It is definitely a chore, but I can see and feel the difference.

Lea O'Neal
Publisher – Welcome Magazine

CHAPTER 1

My Story

I have always eaten a healthy diet, or so I thought. I never believed in diets and ate everything in moderation. I exercised regularly, and when I reached menopause, I believed that adding more soy to my diet would help reduce hot-flashes, mood swings due to a hormonal imbalance, and help prevent osteoporosis because that's what the health magazines and advertisers were telling me.

When I was forty-five, I knew something was wrong because my usual weight of 118-120 pounds climbed to 138 pounds. That started when I was forty-two.

When I would go to the doctor for my annual check-up, I would complain about the way I looked because of the weight gain. My doctor told me I looked great and to compare myself to other women my age and not to women in their thirties. That did make sense to me, but I had a very hard time believing it. When I continued to maintain 138 pounds regardless of what I ate or didn't eat, it took me five years to accept that fact when I turned fifty.

I finally got rid of all my clothes that were size 4's and 6's. I continued to eat the way I always have – everything in moderation – but I added more *soy* including vitamin supplements to my diet because everyone said it was healthy and that the phytoestrogen in soy would improve my hormone balance and hot flashes. I had my soy protein drink in the morning, soy protein bars for a snack, a sandwich for lunch, and a healthy dinner – chicken, fish, beef, vegetables, and/or salads. Sometimes I would just have cereal for dinner.

After eight years. my weight reached 146 pounds. I didn't even weigh that much in my ninth month of pregnancy! I was nauseous, and so uncomfortable all the time, was retaining water (diuretics the doctor prescribed didn't work.) And, I was working out at the gym and playing racquetball three times a week!

In 2003 I began to feel worse! I went to the doctor again and when I stepped on the scale I weighed 148 pounds! The doctor could see I was retaining water, so he ordered extensive blood tests, but the tests showed nothing abnormal.

A week later I had a soy burger for dinner, and when I awoke in the morning, I felt like throwing up. I was weak, anxious, and had diarrhea. I didn't know if I was having a heart attack or if I was going to faint. I asked my husband to bring me the ammonia to sniff while I was lying on the bathroom floor with a damp washcloth on my forehead. I told my husband that my hands felt tingly. I immediately chewed 2 aspirins while he called 911. By the time the ambulance arrived, the episode was subsiding, but I was rushed to the hospital.

While I was in the emergency room, the nurse gave me something to drink then left the room. And, to this day I have no idea what it was. My husband noticed my blood pressure dropping. He immediately called for a nurse – and that's when I had the nurses and doctors running around like chickens without heads! They immediately injected me with epinephrine. What had happened was that I went into anaphylactic shock!

I can't believe that I almost died! It didn't feel like I was dying. I know that if my husband had not been in the room with me at the time, I surely would have died, and the doctors would not have known why. That's pretty scary!

I was put in the intensive care unit for four days hooked up to all kinds of machines. I had three IV's going at the same time, and they started burning because I have small veins and the veins couldn't tolerate the needle indefinitely. The cardiologist inserted a catheter through my neck to monitor my heart to make sure there wasn't any water in the area. At that time they removed the three IV's and placed them in the catheter to my neck. This catheter was very stiff and even the nurse commented that I looked so uncomfortable. She was right!

They ran every test imaginable. The gastroenterologist performed an endoscopy. The endocrinologist ordered a CT scan from my neck to my hips. She said that "carcinoid syndrome" could have the same symptoms as I was showing and was looking for a benign tumor. I had a catheter inserted to perform a 24-hour urine test because they were looking for a bacterial infection. This time when the nurse weighed me I was now 150 pounds! Needless to say, after all the poking, prodding, and blood tests the doctors performed, they didn't find anything – so they said it must have been food poisoning. I told them that I didn't agree because my past experiences with bad food was that I would always throw up if I ate something that didn't agree with me. But as I learned later, food poisoning can in fact cause these symptoms. It's a good thing I didn't eat the food they served in the hospital (I had no appetite), because I would have gone into shock again and really made them crazy! All the food in the hospital has some form of soybean oil or soy flour.

For two weeks, I was afraid to leave the house because since nobody knew what was wrong with me, I didn't know if that would happen again, and I was afraid to drive anywhere. Once I was feeling better, I had my soy protein drink and was out the door. When I got to the parking lot, I started to feel weird again (more like an anxiety attack), but not bad enough to go to the emergency room. I immediately called my husband and he told me to go home and look up "soy allergy" on the Internet. And wouldn't you know it - I had most of the symptoms listed!

I took soy completely out of my diet. After 8 months I was back to 118 pounds. No dieting, no pills, just NO SOY! I am sorry now that I got rid of all those classic gorgeous clothes!

It wasn't easy eliminating soy from my diet. That's because most food products have soy in them. I never realized how many products on the supermarket shelves contain soy. You have to be a wizard to know what the ingredients listed on the label really are. I have to prepare my food from scratch, and I am very limited to eating at restaurants, unless I just have a salad *without* the croutons (They are made from bread, which usually has soy now), I use olive oil and balsamic vinegar, or I bring my own salad dressing. Sure, it's an inconvenience, but I feel so much better physically! And because it's a severe allergy for me, I don't have a choice. That's why I would like to see the restaurants change their food preparation. Never mind the no trans fats! They are made with soybean oil! Now the latest is KFC cooking their chicken in guess what? Soybean oil! And now Dunkin' Donuts are on the bandwagon. That's because they think it's healthier! And now most restaurants and fast food companies are following suit. In the next chapter, I'll get into how this soy allergy has affected my whole life.

You will see that just about everything on the shelf has some form of soy. Ingredients listed are soy flour, soybean oil, lecithin and some vegetable oils. I stay away from vegetable oil that contains soy as well – (they don't tell you that.) I have to be careful with products that have natural flavorings because some of them may contain soy or MSG in it too! Some products will list what the natural flavorings are, which makes it easier for me to decide.

When I am in the store, I pick up an item read the label - put it back on the shelf - move down the aisle pick an item up - put it back on the shelf. It's definitely a chore for me, and very frustrating. Read the labels! You will be amazed at how many products have soy in them! You will see that most products have soybean oil or soy flour. I can't even buy bread off the shelf! So I invested in a Bread Maker that can make two loaves at the same time. Sometimes I just put the Bread Maker on the dough cycle and then I can bake dinner rolls, French bread, etc., in the oven. And if I get lazy, I have finally found various breads I can buy that don't have soy in them at Whole Foods.

I want to add here that it is crucial that I read the labels on everything – including products that I rely on because the manufacturer can change the ingredients.

To give you an example, I always buy the same tomato paste. One day I noticed a new tomato paste from this same manufacturer that included garlic and herbs. I didn't look at the label because I was confident it would be safe. Well, when I was ready to use it, I decided to read the label. Good thing I did! It contained soybean oil! Now why would you need soybean oil when all you are doing is adding garlic and herbs? Be very careful!

To make it even worse, I love chocolate just as much as everyone, but I can't have it! It has lecithin in it and that contains soy too! I don't despair because I do eat ice cream, and I am becoming a better baker! I was never much of a baker before, but I'm learning!

I bake cookies from scratch and chocolate cake substituting Dutch cocoa for the bittersweet chocolate. I haven't perfected the dough crust for pies yet, but I'm working on that. You will find soy-free recipes in Chapter 10.

This is a major food lifestyle change for me, but after four years, I don't feel as deprived as I did in the beginning. I will admit that there are some foods I do miss very much, for instance, Thai food, Japanese food, seafood, and eating at Italian restaurants. Some pizza places make their own dough, but their tomato sauce can have soybean oil in it, or they use vegetable oil in their dough instead of olive oil, and sometimes they don't use real mozzarella cheese. They use a cheese that resembles mozzarella that contains soy and is very stringy. I have called ahead of time to ask about their ingredients because I don't want to be playing Russian roulette. We have a pizza place just up the street from us that makes its own dough from scratch without any soy. In fact, when I went in there, I insisted they show me the can of tomato sauce they use so I could read the label myself. Their sauce was okay, and they use real mozzarella cheese. So these days having pizza is the biggest treat for me. You only have to go into anaphylactic shock once to know you never want that to happen again!

In the beginning I was very frustrated, and sometimes I still get frustrated because soy is not necessary in so many products – it's just cheap filler for the manufacturing companies. Did you know that the soybean industry is over $70 billion dollar a year industry? No wonder the Soybean Industry wants you to believe that soy is so good for you!

I want to share that after about a year of feeling good, I was cooking stir-fry vegetables and decided to try a teaspoon of teriyaki sauce for the flavoring. I was hoping that I had this problem licked. And, what would be the harm with only a teaspoon? Well, surprise!! I had to wake my husband up at 3 am because my throat was closing up! Guess where I was in the middle of the night? You guessed it, the emergency room! I never tried anything like that again.

In April 2007 I had to fly from Atlanta to Ft. Lauderdale. This was the first time I traveled by air since I had discovered my soy allergy. I could take road trips and pack a cooler with three meals per day. But traveling by air is another challenge.

I was so concerned as to what I was going to be able to eat. I packed a half a loaf of bread for sandwiches, baked banana nut bread to bring with me as a snack, and brought nuts. We all know how difficult traveling by air is today because of the strict security. I checked my luggage instead of carrying it on just in case they would throw my food away.

When I arrived, I went to the grocery store and bought

Boar's Head sliced low-sodium ham (this is the only brand that does not have any fillers) and yogurt with the fruit on the bottom. At least breakfast and lunch was taken care of. I knew dinner would be my only problem. Although the hotel I was staying at had a continental breakfast (this breakfast was impressive), they had waffles you could make, donuts, bagels, scrambled eggs, cold cereals, and fruits. I was only able to have the fruit and coffee with half & half – not powdered dairy creamer because it has soybean oil, and the waffles had soy flour in it.

The first night I went to Denny's for dinner (my best choice based on the other restaurants nearby). I was nervous about the menu. I informed the waitress of my soy allergy and decided to order scrambled eggs and told her to have the cook use ONLY butter NO vegetable oil and NO margarine, and cook it in a clean pan. I also told her don't even bother with bringing me toast.

Just to be on the safe side, I took a Benadryl, an antihistamine that blocks histamine receptors and prevents histamine from causing allergic symptoms. That's because my experience in the past has been that I cannot always rely on the cook to know the exact ingredients because like many people, they are not aware that soy is hidden in so many products. Products that say high protein often contain soy flour or other soy derivatives. Vegetable oil also usually contains soybean oil and other derivatives of who knows what, also not listed.

Another significant area that I have to be very careful with is vitamin supplements. Many of them have soy in them but it's not always listed on the label.

Regular multi-vitamins have ingredients such as lecithin, vitamin E (the synthetic type), and would you believe some cellulose (the coating of the capsules) could have soy in it too. My husband had a supplement that he recommended I try. It seemed to be safe, so I tried it. I awoke in the middle of the night and this time I had to use my auto-injector EpiPen (epinephrine) to stop the allergic reaction (the Benadryl wasn't helping this time.) That was the first time I ever had use my EpiPen. You are supposed to go to the hospital after doing this, but I didn't, and I was fine the next day.

Now that I am into reading labels, I don't worry so as much. I have also included buying grass-fed meats whenever possible. All the animals are fed soy, but so far, when I buy meats or chickens in the grocery store, I haven't had any problems. It may seem to you I am going overboard, but it sure is better than going to the hospital again.

In Chapter 9, you will find a list of ingredients that will help you know what to look for.

CHAPTER 2

How My Soy Allergy Affected Me

I n chapter one, I shared my story with you. What I am going to share in this chapter is how having a severe allergy to soy has affected my personal life.

In the beginning, I had no idea what a major lifestyle change this would be. I figured, "Okay, so you won't have protein bars and drinks." Wrong! When I started reading every label on the supermarket shelves, I was shocked at how many of the everyday products we eat have some form of soy. It may be hydrogenated soybean oil, lecithin, soy flour, and sometimes "vegetable oil," unless it states specifically what oils were blended to make it.

I always enjoyed meeting friends for lunch. The first time I ventured out to lunch was to meet a friend at the Olive Garden. I decided to order the soup and salad. I figured this was safe. I questioned the waiter up and down about the ingredients in the minestrone soup, if they bake their bread on the premises, and asked to have them bring me olive oil and vinegar for my salad dressing. I was assured everything was soy free. My friend and I were talking and eating merrily. When we were finished and ready to leave, I started feeling weak and anxious. My friend asked if I was okay, and I wasn't sure, but she said my face looked flushed. I asked for a glass of water so I could take a Benadryl (an anti-histamine). Apparently the waitress didn't understand the severity, so I ran to the bathroom to get the water because I could not wait for her any longer. I didn't want to use my EpiPen because I had never used it before and certainly was unsure how I would react to it. Plus, you're not supposed to take it until symptoms are severe and you are prepared to go to the hospital immediately. I wasn't at that stage. I also took a Xanax for the anxiety, just in case. My friend was so sweet to sit with me until I started feeling better. I made it home okay. I can only assume that it must have been the bread and croutons. So, now I know I can't eat at the Olive Garden.

In another instance similar to the Olive Garden fiasco, my husband and I were invited to an office Christmas party in 2004 at the Outback Steakhouse. I was really nervous about this, but I went through the usual questions and explained my reasons for asking. I knew I couldn't have the "Bloomin' Onions," and I requested that they NOT season my steak with anything except salt and pepper. I also ordered steamed vegetables with no margarine or oil. The bread is shipped frozen and baked on the premises. I have to ask to make sure it does not contain soybean oil or soy flour, so I knew I couldn't have that either. I brought my own salad dressing. Well, no sooner did I finish eating, I had to take the Benadryl again! Could it be that they spray their grill with Pam or some kind of vegetable oil to keep the steaks from sticking? I got through this okay too!

My husband and I love to go out for dinner together. Unfortunately, all that has changed because of my allergy. I have called so many restaurants to find out what their ingredients are, only to be disappointed. So, I have to cook from scratch all the time.

It is a pain in so many ways, like when I was working part time. I had to bring my lunch with me everyday, and then I had to start dinner when I came home. With no occasional meal out and no ordering in, my ritual has become tiresome and boring.

My husband is a member of a literary club that meets once a month for an informal dinner. Everyone brings a covered dish, and the club orders fried chicken and biscuits. I bring a big spring salad mix garnished with chickpeas, olives, mushrooms, tomatoes, and mandarin oranges mixed with my salad dressing. Everyone loves it, but that's all I can eat! For years I could never understand why I was always so nauseous when we came home. Now I know why – it was the soy. Sometimes, I don't even bother going because I feel so isolated. During the year they have ceilidhs and other Scottish parties that are catered, and I can't eat anything at all! So, once again, I have to eat before we go.

In chapter one, I have already described my recent experience when traveling by air. Now I want to share my experience as it relates to weekend getaways.

We were visiting my husband's aunt in Tennessee. It's a tradition in this family that when we get together, we all go to the BBQ restaurant. This is a small town where everybody knows each other. I knew for sure I wouldn't be able to eat a thing, so we packed a cooler for me with breakfast, lunch and dinner. I felt so pathetic having to eat my sandwich out of the trunk of the car in the parking lot of the restaurant before we joined the family already seated inside. I was only able to order coffee to feel like I was joining in with everyone. How frustrating is that?

The first few years of our marriage, New Orleans was a favorite get-away for us. Jambalaya, crawfish pie, and filé gumbo! The best eating in the world – cheap and plenty of it! Oh well, no Café du Monde for me. No Cajun food at Mulate's. No Café Sbisa. No popping into

Café Pontalba on Jackson Square. No hole-in-the-wall surprises for red beans and rice. What's left? Well, there's a funky coffee shop near the equally funky French Market where I love to shop. My husband loves the used bookstores. We always find art to buy on Royal Street. But to be surrounded by great places to eat and not being able to eat carefree, why bother?

This allergy can be very debilitating. I recently read that once you develop a severe allergy, the fear of an allergic reaction happening again never leaves you! At one point, my husband was concerned that I would end up with an anxiety disorder because of it. I don't have an anxiety disorder, but for me the initial symptoms of anaphylactic shock start off as an anxiety attack and that is why it's difficult to decipher. For example, whether I'm experiencing an allergic reaction, or I'm afraid I'm going to have an allergic reaction, my heart begins to race. I feel slight chest pain, shortness of breath, nausea, weak and light-headed, fear of dying, and chills or hot flushes. Now you understand what I have to deal with on a daily basis.

For example, on the way to Grandfather Mountain in North Carolina for the Scottish Highland Games, we stopped at a Waffle House to get something to eat. After explaining my allergy, I ordered scrambled eggs made in butter, they told me the grits were made with butter and not margarine. I was so worried that I made myself throw up before we left. I was afraid to believe that the meal was prepared just for me. After we were driving for a few minutes, I started having an anxiety attack and wanted my husband to drive us home, even though we were half way to North Carolina – once again, I took a Xanax to try and calm myself down. He told me not to worry and take deep slow breaths and hold them for eight seconds. I did that and was feeling better.

I'm learning to live with this allergy because my husband and I went back to Grandfather Mountain last year for the Highland Games. We filled our cooler with yogurt, hard-boiled eggs, dinner, nuts to snack on, and my banana nut bread so I wouldn't starve to death. I couldn't eat anything served at the Games. There was one evening we were going with a few other couples to a very nice place for dinner. I knew in advance what restaurant it was because a reservation was made. I called them way in advance gave my name and the party I would be with. Asked a lot of questions about their menu. They were very gracious, made a notation, and when we showed up, the Maitre de asked is Dianne Gregg here? I introduced myself and he said not to worry because the servers were aware of my problem. Our server was great! The chef made everything just for me! I enjoyed this meal so much, but it was also a fortune (well worth it), even though I couldn't eat the bread.

We participate in the Highland Games in Stone Mountain, Georgia, every year. We have a tent set up with food and beverages for members and guests of the MacGregor Clan. I bring a separate sandwich for myself and various foods that everyone likes to eat, including snacks and desserts. I especially used to like the hot cocoa that is available at the hospitality booth for sponsors. For years I would mix their hot cocoa and coffee. Well, now that I'm in the habit of reading labels, I can't even have the hot cocoa or the powdered dairy creamer for my coffee! They both have soybean oil or soy lecithin. Who would have thought?

Now I will discuss the effects when it comes to my business life and the limitations that have been a major concern for me.

For so many years I was always active in many business organizations networking with various people to build my photography business. I was a board member on almost all of them. We met monthly for luncheons and listened to speakers, or we held promotional and charitable events. Well, now I don't go to any of them because I can't eat the food. Why pay money for luncheons or dinner events just to sit there when I can't eat anything? When I have inquired in the past regarding the menus, they aren't sure what they are, and when I do put in a special order for something, I'm afraid that it could be cross-contaminated with the very ingredient I MUST stay away from.

There are so many people who don't know what they are eating or preparing. Even I didn't know before this allergy hit me, and I was forced to read every label and understand the hidden names of the listed ingredients with everything I use.

For example, I attended a networking group that was followed by a wonderful looking buffet. I asked to speak to the chef of the catering company. The chef had the menu in hand and searched for possibilities for me to eat. He recommended the grilled chicken that was only seasoned with lemon. This sounded interesting and I was smart enough to ask "do you spray the grill with vegetable oil?" The chef replied "yes", so I couldn't have the chicken either. I stayed for a little while to mingle with others, and then I left.

Once I attended an evening event that had a Mexican-food-only buffet. It's a good thing I ate before I left the house. In the business arena I really feel isolated. And this makes me feel out of the loop from many of the things I have always enjoyed doing.

It's the same thing when I get invited to parties. I'm grateful that my friends are very thoughtful and considerate of my allergy and try very hard to have food that I can eat. I always bring my wonderful spring salad with my dressing on it. Everybody loves it, and so I buy the dressing for all my friends so they can have it in their pantry. It's funny—some guests bring food and one of my friends gives them the third degree! While I'm there listening to the ingredients saying okay, okay, and then bam! The last ingredient I can't have! Then my friend makes sure I know what I can and can't have!

Another friend had her 50th birthday party and made sure everything was soy-free. There were some fried coconut chicken fingers appetizers. I asked the server what kind of oil it was fried in. She called the caterer just to make sure it wasn't fried in vegetable oil. It wasn't—so I ate only one. I can never be sure unless I prepare something myself, but I was fine that night. I've never been a control freak, but you can't take chances with a life-and-death situation!

Another place I can eat is the Ritz Carlton! It was another friend's birthday that I had the opportunity to eat there, and of course I called and let them know my situation and whose event I was attending. I have to tell you, I was very impressed. As soon as everyone was seated, the restaurant manager came up to me and said they had a meeting regarding the event and that my name came up. He wanted to reassure me that every waiter there knew my situation. At the end of the meal, the general manager approached me and asked if everyone took good care of me. I told him I had a wonderful meal and that everyone was great! By the way, the Ritz Carlton only uses peanut oil. Whether you just go to the Ritz Carlton to eat or stay as a guest, they are worth every penny they charge.

When it comes to supplements, I have to be very careful. I have to order a special blend multi-vitamin that has no soy whatsoever. After I was taking it for a few weeks, I started feeling weak and nauseous. The site I purchased it from checked with the doctor that makes it and there isn't anything in it to make me feel that way, so I started taking it again. It must have been my nervousness about trying something new.

Atlanta is growing by leaps and bounds and more and more restaurants are opening up. Unfortunately, to my disappointment, they use soybean oil. Bummer!

As you can imagine, this is not an easy lifestyle when it comes to food.

The good thing is that it inspired me to write this book and do my research about soy so I can pass this information on to you. Now you will be informed and decide for yourself. Based on the information in the following chapters, do you really want to take a chance and harm your health, or do you want to heal in a natural way?

One opinion I have for women when they are trying diets such as Jenny Craig or NutriSystem is I'm sure it's made with soybean oil or soy flour. But think of this—aren't they already prepared in smaller portions? Why can't you do that on your own? Because of what happened to me, I believe that all of these foods with soy contribute to the weight gain, water retention, and bloating. Although mine is a more serious case, why else would I have lost all that weight so quickly and kept it off? I may not be able to eat all of the same foods as before, but when I cook from scratch, I can eat everything from meat, stews, casseroles, chicken, fish, pasta, bread, all vegetables, and fruits, cookies, cake, and ice cream, and nuts. And, I'm still 116-118 pounds!

So, even though I'm frustrated that I can't eat wherever I want, I'm healthier because of it. But there's so much more to the soy story than soy allergy and what it has put me through. Do you want to possibly risk having a problem with your thyroid that would require you to be on medication for the rest of your life? How about if you are a cancer survivor? Do you want to risk promoting new tumors? Do you want to hurt your infant with soy formula, risk early puberty in girls, or breasts in your boys? No? Then read on!

CHAPTER 3

Another Woman's Story

Here is another compelling story I read online and thought it deserved it's own chapter.

This is my true story, nothing altered. These are facts as they relate to my experience, and my opinions based on what I have read and feel. I am relating them to warn other young health-conscious women who are unwittingly harming themselves and so what I am going through has some purpose. It would make what I have gone through worth something and not in vain.

In 1989 I graduated from high school in a small town in Texas and couldn't wait to hit the big college city so I could begin to live my own life. One of the changes I wanted to make was to eat healthier. My family wasn't big on tofu, yogurt, or fruits. I also didn't want to gain the freshman 15. Once I moved to health-conscious Austin, Texas, with its parks, hike and bike trails, and health food stores, I began to fortify my body with the best and healthiest foods I could find. Tofu was the main ingredient in every healthy dish, and I bought soymilk almost every day because it was better than milk, or so I thought. I used it for everything from cereal to smoothies or just to drink for a quick snack. I bought soy muffins, miso soup with tofu, soybeans, soybean sprouts, etc. All the literature in all the health and fitness magazines said that soy protected you against everything from heart disease to breast cancer. It was the magical isoflavones, it was the estrogen-like hormones that all worked to help you stay young and healthy

But I wasn't that healthy. I looked great, I was working out all the time, but my menstrual cycle was off. At 20 I started taking birth control pills to regulate my menstrual cycle. One brand would work for a few months but then I would become irregular again. The doctors kept switching the brands and assuring me that I'd find the one that would work. In addition to this I began to suffer from painful periods. I began to get puffy—not fat, I wasn't gaining weight, just getting rounder. It was as though I was losing my muscle tone. I wasn't looking as good as I had before, despite all my exercising. I began to suffer from fits of depression and get hot flashes. I mistook all this for PMS since my periods were irregular. I had no way of knowing when I was going to begin my period.

Now, I had started using soy when I was 19. The onset of these problems quickly began at 20. By the time I was 25 my periods were so bad I couldn't walk. The birth control pills never made them regular or less painful so I decided to stop taking them. I went on like this for another two years until I realized my pain wasn't normal. In 1998, when I was 27 years old, my gynecologist found two cysts in my uterus. Both were the size of tennis balls. I was scared to death! I went through surgery to have them removed and thank God, they were benign. The gynecologist told me to go back on birth control pills. I didn't. In 1998, he discovered a lump in my breast. Again, I went through surgery and again it was benign.

It was in November 2000 that my glands swelled up and my gums became inflamed. Thinking I had a tooth infection, I went to the dentist who told me that my teeth were not the problem. After a dose of antibiotics, the swelling still did not go down. At this point, I could feel a tiny nodule on the right side of my neck. No one else could feel it. I told my mother I had thyroid trouble. This was based only on a hunch. She, along with others in my family, said I was being silly. No one in the family suffered from thyroid trouble. "What's a thyroid?" was what my friends would say.

Going on a hunch, I saw a specialist who diagnosed me with Papillary Thyroid Carcinoma. After a series of tests, he told me it was cancer. My fiancé and I sat stunned. I was dreading another operation but so far, every lump had been benign. We were not prepared and I was so scared. We scheduled surgery right away. The specialist told us that it would only be after the operation that a pathologist would be able to tell us for sure if it was cancer. They found a tumor on my right lobe composed of irregular cells and another smaller tumor growing on the left, so the entire thyroid was removed. No harm was done to my vocal chords, no harm to my parathyroid, but I now had an ugly scar and would be dependent on thyroid hormones the rest of my life. They told me that after undergoing radioactive iodine I would be safe and assured me that I could live a long life.

After treatment, I began to search for the cause of all these problems. An x-ray I had done at age 8 was under suspicion, as was stress—everything got blamed on stress, genes, maybe that time I tried to smoke a cigarette (I was never a smoker but tried once), maybe that summer when I was 25 and began to drink vodka and to try mixed drinks (I was never one for alcohol, but wanted to know what the hype was about). I began to look for esoteric reasons like not being spiritual enough. I never once thought it could be all the soy I had consumed for nearly ten years. After all, soy is healthy. I never drank soft drinks, and even when I was under excruciating pain, never took aspirin or headache medications. Maybe it was birth control pills.

I came upon a Web page that linked thyroid problems to soy intake and the conspiracy of soy marketed as a health food when in fact it is only a toxic by-product of the vegetable oil industry. This was insane, I thought. After all, the health and fitness magazines had said nothing about soy being harmful. I visited an herbalist who was diagnosed with thyroid cancer in 1985. She informed me that soy was the culprit. She was a health-conscious individual who in her twenties fortified her diet with soy. A few years after that, she had to have a hysterectomy due to cysts and other uterine problems. A few months later, I met another acquaintance that had consumed soy and had thyroid cancer. She was 27 years old! I met a girl from England through the Internet in a thyroid cancer forum, had just undergone surgery and she was only 19 years old! What was going on? The research said that thyroid cancer was more common in older women; age 50 years old or older. It was said to be genetic or the result of nuclear fallout like in Chernobyl.

I met another acquaintance who is also a health-conscious individual that just found out she has thyroid cancer and she was also only 29 years old. I searched the Internet and found breast cancer linked to the radioactive iodine given during treatment. This didn't seem true. As fearful as I am of anything nuclear, the treatment has been given for over 150 years. Breast cancer is linked to estrogen. What mimics estrogen in the female body? SOY! I am not a scientist or a doctor but I know my body. I knew that there were changes going on and I did search for clues as to why, but I never suspected soy because until now I never once found a single article that stated soy could be dangerous. Evening primrose oil I heard taken in large amounts, vitamin A, C, and E could make tumors grow if taken in large dosages. MSG, even tuna is harmful but never once mentioned SOY. Women who took soy before thyroid problems will continue to eat it because they are not aware of what soy actually does, what it contains, and how it reacts in the female body. I think this is the reason that women with thyroid cancer often develop breast cancer later.

Now it all makes sense. If you trace the problems I have had, they are all related to hormones. Taking birth control pills I believe only added more hormones to my body that I didn't need. I believe it was eating fruit, and veggies, no smoking, no drinking, and exercising, that kept my first surgeries benign. I wasn't as lucky the last time.

My co-worker is big into soy and I see her losing hair and gaining weight despite a walking workout during her break and after work, and apples and oranges for lunch. She just had cysts removed from her uterus too. I warn her to stay off the soy. I refer her to Web sites but until it is on the evening news on all major networks, women will suffer. I say what I can, but at the Christmas potluck, every dish contained soy in one form or another. It's now the staple of the new American diet—eat right, eat for health, eat to ward off cancer, AND IT'S SOY!

In 1994, I had my thyroid-stimulating hormone (TSH) checked again on a hunch. I was suffering from lethargic days, fits of depression, feeling off, and mild digestive problems. My TSH was a 6. A good physician, taking into account my symptoms, would have explored this. We are not always blessed with good physicians. Many don't know what a thyroid gland is, what it does or even where it is, and they miss important signs.

By the way, today I have normal periods even though I am not on birth control pills. Even though I have had to change my dosage of thyroid hormone since the thyroidectomy, I have not touched soy for two years.

Dear readers, please use my story in any way you can. There are so many young girls consuming soy because they think they are taking care of themselves and want to be healthy. It is so unfair that the information about the dangers of soy isn't more widely circulated. It is sad. Health is wealth and until 1998 no matter how badly things went—car breaking down, bills, and bad dates—I felt comforted in that I had my health. So many people feel this way.

It is a terrible blow when you realize you are not as healthy as you thought and that the information that you depended on was wrong.[1]
Tera

" I am a 58-year-old woman, and have had two operations for cancer. The first operation was for uterine cancer, the second for a tumor growing on the abdominal wall, which was possibly caused by breakage of the uterus in the first operation. At any rate, the OBGYN that performed my first op. wanted me to take the combo estrogen/progesterone drug...I opted to take phytoestrogens and use a progesterone cream. When I found cancer once again, I went to an iconologist (I believe, a very responsible one). He immediately told me to get off soy, black cohosh, and any other estrogenic substance that I had been taking. He then put me on a large dose of progesterone. I am doing very well, staying on progesterone for the time-being, and treating any estrogenic property like the plague."[2]

"*I am a 68-year-old woman who now has hypothyroidism and alopecia from taking soy products. After being taken off HRT, I got uretheritis, vaginal dryness, and thrush. My GP prescribed Estriol cream and suggested that eating soy would help redress the estrogen deficiency. For several months, I put about 5oz of Soymilk on my cereals. I hated the taste so when I saw an advertisement for Soy Isoflavone capsules I thought them a good alternative. I took the recommended dose which I now calculate contained 36mg Daidzein and 9mg Genistein per day and other isoflavones. The advertising is so convincing that it never occurred to me to question the products' safety. After a few weeks of taking the capsules, I experienced nausea. After about three months of taking the capsules my hair began to come out .A month later I was rapidly balding. My doctor started a series of blood tests, which indicated alopecia, autoimmune disease, and hypothyroidism. I read an article in a magazine warning of the side effects of soy products. I told my doctor and we started to look at the symptoms from a different perspective. After five weeks since I stopped taking the capsules my facial hair, eyebrows and pubic hair are slowly growing. I do not know whether I will regain all the hair that I have lost or whether my thyroid function will ever return to normal I only know that Soy products are dangerous and should be banned.*" [3]

[1] http://www.the7thfire.com/health_and nutrition/soydangers.htm
[2_3] Testimonial courtesy of http://www.soyonline.com.nz

CHAPTER 4

An Athlete's Story

Here is a story that was provided by SoyOnline.com.nz from a professional baseball player, and testimonials.

I am a former professional athlete - who was fed soy formula as a baby (born in 1954) due to an allergy to my Mother's breast milk. I have become very interested in Alternative Medicine - and I have just recently started to read about the negative effects that soy formula can have on people for their entire life. The more I read - the more of my own personal circumstances become explainable. And the explanation points to having been fed soy formula as a baby.

Growing up I was always a good athlete - and I was always big. The first time I ever remember going on a diet was when I was 12 years old. I weighed 160 lbs - and they wanted me to play on a football team in my town. The age of most players was 13 and 14 - and they had a weight limit of 130 lbs. For six weeks, I ate just lean protein and salads - and I ran miles and miles on top of going to football practice every day. I got down to 138 lbs and could not lose another pound. That was the start of my life long battle against my own weight - and what my weight meant as I pursued my athletic career.

I always carried extra weight despite being very active and eating small amounts of "good for you" type foods. For years I consumed no sugars - no candy etc...

During my high school years - I was an all-state basketball and baseball player. I graduated from high school at 6' 4" and weighing about 220 lbs. I went to college on an athletic scholarship - and constantly had to monitor my weight, to keep it under 235 lbs. I used to fast (just drank water) for two and three days at a time - despite doing all of the running and working out that these sports required. At the end of college, the Baltimore Orioles Major League Baseball team drafted me. At that point, in my life I weighed 240 lbs

When I started my professional baseball career, I was told I had a weight problem and that I had to do extra running etc. to get my weight down. My weight always stayed at about 245 lbs unless, I went on starvation/liquid protein diets. As I continued my baseball career - I continued to battle my weight, despite everything that I did.

In 1978 during the off-season I was working out at a gym and one of the guys working out there was in med school. He knew who I was and he knew how hard I was working out. He said that he could not imagine that I was going home and stuffing myself with donuts and beer. And, that based on what I was doing he thought that my weight should be in the neighborhood of 195 lbs to 205 lbs. He said that he wanted to run some tests on my body and have me keep a food and exercise diary for six weeks I said okay.

For the next 6 weeks, I maintained my program: Full court basketball games each morning from 10:00 am to 12 noon. Weigh lifting for 45 minutes, followed by a four-mile jog. And then more full court basketball from 3:30 to 5:30 pm. I would eat a bowl of corn flakes for breakfast - no lunch - and a regular dinner, no dessert and no snacks. They weighed me and took my body fat percentages in a water tank that was suppose to be precise.

At the end of the six weeks, the people from the University of Pennsylvania told me that they had good news and bad news for me. The bad news was that my body is functioning at a slower rate than most other people. Which meant that I would always be big, and would always have to watch what I ate, and that I could never ever stop exercising or I would blow up like a blimp. The good news was that because I was "going slower" than other people - a lot of the signs of aging that affect other people would impact me at a later point in my life than most people are affected

Well I am almost 54 years old and my hair is still all dark brown with very few grays - my skin has absolutely no wrinkles - and people think I am in my early 40's! I also have fulfilled the other part of what I was told 30 years ago - I am a big guy standing 6'4" and weighing 330 lbs I have to watch everything I eat and I work out 5 to 6 days every week.

Thyroid tests come back as normal, I am told I have a slow metabolism. Somehow, I think that having been fed nothing but soy formula for the first 18 months of my life may have contributed to this.

Thanks for the chance to voice this.

Rowland George

"My son recently had his thyroid removed at the age of 33 with a diagnosis of Follicular Cancer. As an infant, he was fed soy formula and still uses soymilk on his cereal. He recently had a head CT scan for a medical reason and an incidental finding was that his brain is undersized. He has normal to above normal intelligence. I read on your website that this is related to soy as well. I was a very nutritionally aware mother and I am shocked to find that he may have been harmed by soy formula. I thought I was doing what was best because he cried and had intestinal discomfort on milk."

I'm a 31 year old Australian male in reference to thyroid problems, I think there is a high chance that my soy consumption (2-4 liters/week used as alternative to cow's milk) over the last 5 or more years, has led to my hypothyroid condition (Hashimotos disease), discovered just this year. The thyroid anti-bodies were about 60 times higher than normal and of course, TSH high and thyroxine low. I now have to take thyroxin tablets for the rest of my life, and this has brought the TSH and thyroxin levels back to normal."

"I have been on Atkins for three months and have been increasing my soy consumption hand over fist. I am a true athlete and teach classes 5 days a week. In this last month, I have not felt very well. I was eating two Atkins bars a day, an Atkins shake, an Atkins bag of chips, and Todd's bagels. Wow! I could not believe the total - perhaps 80 grams of soy. Now it's over! I feel that the risk is real and the negative side affects are because of the Soy. I only wish I read this a month ago. This really freaked me out that I will never consume soy ever again!"

CHAPTER 5

Soy Background

Soy has been used for food for humans and animals for thousands of years. Eaten occasionally in small quantities and properly prepared, it has been a minor but useful food in East Asia. How did soy change from being a good food to being a dangerous one? A few pioneers have told the story better than I can.[1,2,3,4,5] I want to give you an idea of what I've learned from them. Except as noted, this chapter is from their writings, which you can easily find using the chapter endnotes.

The Chinese first used soybeans and soy straw and leaves for human and animal consumption four thousand years ago or more. The oldest Chinese writings about soy are found in a 7th century BC collection of poems and songs from the Western Zhou dynasty (11th to 8th century BC). [6,7] However, in Japan and China, soy is not used as a replacement for animal products. I keep reading that Asians get a lot of their protein from soy, but that's not true. One study says that Chinese traditionally got less than 2 percent of their calories from soy and 65 percent from pork, with the Japanese getting a similar amount from fish instead of pork. They eat more natural products. Their meat is less fatty and they eat more fish and vegetables. Their diets are lower in chemicals and toxins because they eat less processed foods.

At some point the Chinese realized that there were bad side affects from what we know today to be anti-nutrients or soy toxins. They developed ways of removing toxins, such as in the traditional Chinese way of making soymilk. They first soaked and partially sprouted the beans and then ground them into mush using lots of water. They put the mush into a cloth bag and squeezed out some of the toxins along with the water. Then they boiled what was left in fresh water. They discarded the scum that rose to the top, which got rid of even more toxins.

Today's fast, cheap way of making soybeans "edible" does not remove the soy toxins and may contain some new ones. The pre-soaking step is shorter, and the scum is not removed, so the soy toxins stay in. The commercial way is to cook the soy paste in a pressure cooker, which can destroy some of the nutrition. Also, even though soybeans contain some omega-3 fatty acids, high temperature and pressure can cause the fatty acids to go bad, that is, to become rancid. Some researchers think that the commercial process may even introduce carcinogens.[8,9] (I got some of this info from two FDA scientists!)

The soy industry chose profits over disposal by expanding the market and finding more ways to use soy ingredients. They could only feed animals a certain amount before they developed health problems. It was clear that the toxic effects of the natural toxins in soy were not being removed from the finished products for animal and human consumption. Adverse biological effects were well documented. The trypsin inhibitors interfere with digestion that can lead to gastric distress, poor protein digestion, and an overworked pancreas.[10] The efforts to remove the toxins were abandoned as being technically difficult and expensive. Because of these toxins, soy protein was never given GRAS (Generally Regarded as Safe) status. The carcinogenic risks remain to this day.

In 1988 a series of industry conferences was arranged in the Netherlands entitled "Anti-nutritional Factors in

Legume Seeds," and numerous scientists presented research that shows that soy and other leguminous seed feeds are toxic to animal species and that it is economically impractical to remove them. Much more heat processing to remove some toxins would destroy the protein, making it useless as a food.[11]

From the landfill to your kitchen, soy protein, and other sludge is left over from the oil extraction. Since 1950 there has been an explosive growth of processed foods, and many contained soy oil, especially vegetable oil, margarine, and shortening. Soy lecithin is used as an emulsifier. After a while, the soy industry got the idea of using the waste for animal feed instead of dumping it. Then the industry decided to promote it for human consumption. At first soy protein was promoted as a cheap meat extender for the poor or the budget conscious. The real breakthroughs came when the industry began touting it as a great source of protein for vegetarians and then as a miracle health food for everyone.

They convinced a more affluent society to pay more for soy-based imitation foods. That's how they began to sell soy products to the health conscious as a "miracle" product that would prevent heart disease, cancer, hot flashes, and osteoporosis. Instead of a poverty food, it's now nearly as expensive as meat, and pricier than dairy.

Advertising articles in magazines promote soy as the "health food." Easily recognizable soy foods such as tofu and soymilk, as well as meat and dairy alternatives such as tofu hot dogs, burgers and soy cheeses, are beginning to show up on many household grocery shopping lists. In fact, retail sales of soy food products reached $1.1 billion dollars in1996 (the most recent year for which data are available), compared to just $300 million in 1980, according to information compiled by Soyatech, Inc., a research and consulting firm in Bar Harbor, Maine. During that same period, sales of tofu increased from $37 million to $144 million, while soymilk sales rocketed from just $1.5 million to $124 million![12]

The U.S. Market 2007, published by Soyatech, Inc. and SPINS list soy food sales from 1992 - 2006 with an increase from $300 million to $3.9 billion. Between 2005 and 2006 there was a 1.4% increase in overall soy foods sales. This represents a general leveling off of sales, but some categories, like soymilk, have experienced greater growth and others such as energy bars have not.[13]

The soybean industry has come a long way because they have now identified us as the "health conscious" and promote soy as nutritious. With affluent, health-conscious buyers, so what had been trash became a goldmine.

Now the soy industry has found another way to make soy products even less healthy—and are upsetting the ecology and the economics of farming to boot. In 1997 Argentina became one of the first countries to use Monsanto's genetically modified (GM) seed. Monsanto has gained millions in profits from sales of its popular herbicide, Roundup/Æ. Soy is of course among those "Roundup-Ready/Æ" crops. The bacteria died, and dead weeds would not rot. Being resistant to this powerful herbicide, farmers are able to spray more of it on their crops, resulting in higher levels of toxins in the harvested product. Recent studies have shown that sprayed soybean crops have an elevated estrogen level that is much higher than the soybean's already high levels. Farmers and neighbors near the GM fields suffered health problems such as rashes and tearing eyes, and many livestock died or gave birth to deformed young. More land was leveled for more soy production, and the big farmers drove small farmers off their land. The production of other staples to feed the people of Argentina fell and was replaced by soybeans grown for export to Europe and China.

Instead of being an exporter, China is now the world's largest importer of U.S. soy products used for human consumption as well as meal for poultry, swine, and fish industries. DuPont, the world's largest producer of soy protein, owns 20 joint ventures and independent investment enterprises in China, with a total investment of more than $700 million.

From a simple food used in moderation in ancient China, soybeans have grown into a toxic tsunami. Soy products are now so widespread that it is going to be hard for us to find high ground to avoid the effects of this tidal wave.

[1] Jones, J. (2002, October 6). Dangers of isoflavones in soy and soy-based foods. Retrieved July 19, 2007, from Web site:
http://www.rense.com/general30/soye.htm

[2] Farr, G. (2003, January 22). Concerns regarding soybeans. Retrieved April 5, 2007, from Web site: http://www.becomehealthynow.com/article/soy/1090/
This Web page also gives access to other Farr articles used in this chapter: "Just How Much Soy Did Asians Eat?" and "Soy: Too Good to Be True."

[3] Fallon, S. (2000, March) The ploy of soy. *Consumer Health Organization of Canada, 23*(3). Retrieved June, 2, 2007, from Web site:
http://www.consumerhealth.org/articles/display.cfm?ID=20000501001338

[4] Fallon, S. A., & Enig, M. G. (2000, April-May). Tragedy and hype: The Third International Soy Symposium. *Nexus Magazine, 7*(3). Retrieved April 17, 2007, from http://www.nexusmagazine.com/articles/soydangers.html

[5] Daniel, K. T. (2005). *The whole soy story: The dark side of America's favorite health food.* Washington, DC: New Trends Publishing, Inc.

[6] Gai, J., & Guo. W. (n.d) History of maodou [immature soybean] production in China. Document from Nanjing Agricultural University. Retrieved August 17, 2007, from Asian Vegetable Research and Development Center Web site: http://www.avrdc.org/pdf/soybean/gaipresentation.pdf

[7] China Culture (2003). Western Zhou Dynasty. Retrieved August 17, 2007, from Web site: http://www.chinaculture.org/gb/en_aboutchina/2003-09/24/content_22699.htm

[8] Doerge, D., & Sheehan, D. (1999). Letter to FDA. Retrieved July 14, 2007, from http://preterhuman.net/texts/other/SoyFacts.doc

[9] Henkel, J. (2000, May-June). Soy: Health claims for soy protein, questions about other components. *FDA Consumer Magazine.* Retrieved July 15, 2007, from http://www.fda.gov/fdac/features/2000/300_soy.html

[10] Rackis, Joseph J. et al., "The USDA trypsin inhibitor study.

[11] Sainsi, H. S., Huisman, J., Poel, T. F. B., van der, & Liener, I. E. (Eds.) (1989). Legume seed oligosaccarides [Abstract]. Proceedings of the First International Workshop on "Antinutritional Factors (ANF) in Legume Seeds", November 23-25, 1988, Wageningen, Netherlands. 1989, 329-341. Retrieved August 28, 2007, from http://www.infoharvest.ca/pcd/dbabs.cgi?rnum=89

[12] http://soyfoods.com/SANA/index.html retrieved October 19, 2007

[13] http://www.soyfoods.org/products/sales-and-trends/

Source: *Soyfoods: The U.S. Market 2007*, published by Soyatech, Inc. and SPINS, Retrieved October 17, 2007

CHAPTER 6

Soybean Industry in America

W hen it comes to soy, there are strong financial incentives by companies like Monsanto, Cargill Foods, Soylife, and the many soybean councils that represent the agribusinesses who grow this crop. Soy is cheap and very profitable. The production of soybeans is 40 times more now than it was starting in the 20th century. This is why the soybean industry concentrated on finding alternative uses and new markets for soybeans.

"Soy Serves Up Healthy Benefits" will get your attention. It made me a believer through health magazines and the media advertising such as those sponsored by the Indiana Soybean Alliance of the Indiana Soybean Board.[1]

There was considerable research done since WW II about the harmful substance within the soybean.

Soy contains several naturally occurring compounds that are toxic to humans and animals. The soy industry frequently refers to these toxins as anti-nutrients, which implies that they somehow act to prevent the body from getting the complete nutrition it needs from a food. The soy toxins (such as phytic acid) can certainly act in this manner, but they also have the ability to target specific organs, cells and enzyme pathways, and their effects can be devastating. As with any toxin, there will be a dose at which negative effects are not observed.

By 1985, there was a considerable body of research from U.S. Government and university laboratories and British government institutions warning of the health dangers of soy foods, particularly to high-risk consumers such as infants and vegetarian women. These were published in scientific journals. In response, in 1985 the soy processing industry in the U.S. held a number of conferences and devised a program, "Soy 2000," the intent of which was to aggressively promote soy as a health food when they already knew it contained biologically active levels of toxins. This involved heavy political lobbying of Congress and Federal regulators, a vast advertising program, planting favorable articles in popular and academic media, obtaining huge Federal farming subsidies, and sponsorship of meetings by the U.S Department of Agriculture. The aim of Soy 2000 was to promote to the consumers that soy was a proven health food with no adverse effects. Their claim was that millions of Asians have been consuming soy in large quantities for thousands of years and are all remarkably healthy as a result. American consumers were expected to believe this, and most of us did! Another line of the Soy 2000 campaign was that scientists who performed research that was unfavorable to soy were persecuted, ridiculed, and libeled. They lost research funds and had their research reports watered down or refused outright by the editors of academic journals. Some Federal scientists have had their laboratories closed down.[2]

With innovative technologies, pioneering research and development partnerships, food and beverage manufacturers now have a never-before-seen opportunity to capitalize on the boom in the wellness food marketplace by creating new soy inclusive products to meet today's evolving health-conscious consumer.

Did you catch that? Never-before-seen opportunity to

capitalize on the boom! What has already begun is the Soy 2020 vision check-off by the United Soybean Board (USB). This is a board made up of 64 members of farmer-leaders acting on behalf of the 680,000 U.S. soybean farmers that "invests in research, promotion, marketing and commercialization programs to help expand and develop markets for U.S. soybeans. As part of the check-off program, every soybean farmer contributes a 0.5 percent of the market price for each bushel sold. These funds are used at the state level by qualified state soybean boards (QSSBs) and nationally by USB to support the goals of U.S. soybean farmers in six main areas: animal utilization, industrial utilization, human utilization, supply, industry relations and market access."[3]

In March 2006, Monsanto approached USB to undergo this visioning process to bring together all facets of the U.S. soybean industry. The objective was to create a vision for the future of U.S. soybeans that would be a collaboration to drive success for soybeans despite what the future may hold. USB quickly brought on additional financial sponsorships with a contribution of its own, as well as support pledged from Monsanto, Deere and Company, the National Oilseed Processors Association and Farm Credit Council.

"Soy 2020 is a great example of the different players in the soybean industry coming together for a common goal," says Ernesto Fajardo, vice president of U.S. crop business for Monsanto. "The established vision of Soy 2020 will allow a proactive, nimble approach to optimizing the U.S. soybean industry in the future."[4]

By the year 2020, the world population will most likely exceed 8 billion people, with 93 percent of growth taking place in developing countries. Continued population growth, combined with an increasing economic status in developing countries, will require a global effort to feed a hungry world and provide the energy required to sustain global economic growth.

They say that the soybean value chain should promote soy health and nutrition benefits, environmental sustainability and technology safety to global consumers of food, fuel, and feed, as well as support the viability and growth of animal agriculture, renewable energy, and other soy-consuming industries. The policy frameworks will be undertaken by the American Soybean Association.[5]

So, while they are promoting health and nutrition to consumers, they want to enable soybean farmers to gain access into new markets, including plastics, lubricants, coatings, printing inks, adhesives, and other specialty products. They are trying to build demand for new soy products to consumers. Maybe because they are afraid that the consumers will finally learn the truth and not buy food products with soy in them! I can only hope.

Ashland Chemical introduced five new lines of soy resins under the ENVIREZ name increasing the use of soy in their product lines. The new line of soy resins will be incorporated into applications such as the new model tractor hoods for both John Deere and Case New Holland. Even the Ford Motor Company has announced a breakthrough in soy-based polyurethane foams, a primary substance that makes up a vehicle's seat cushions, seat backs, armrests, and head restraints.[6] If a product like soy has so many uses, this does concern me. Since I have a potentially fatal soy allergy, will I have to watch what I touch, drive, and sit down on as well as what I eat?

Now, do you see what a big business this is?

[1] Galeaz, K. (n.d.) Soy serves up healthy benefits. Retrieved May 1, 2007, from two Indiana Soybean Alliance Web sites: http://www.soybean.org/health.html and http://www.indianasoybeanboard.com/radio/index.shtml
[2] James, R. (2007, August 15). Personal communication from Soyonline Organization: http://www.soyonline.com.nz
[3] Latest from the Soybean Checkoff. (2007). Retrieved August 20, 2007, from Web site: http://unitedsoybean.org/Media/Default.aspx
[4] Soybean Checkoff Takes Lead in Visioning to 2020 (2007, March 2). Retrieved April 17, 2007, from Web site: Soybean Checkoff Takes Lead in Visioning to 2020
[5] Soy 2020. (n.d.) Retrieved March 6, 2007, from Web site: http://www.soy2020vision.com/
[6] Checkoff Helps Introduce First Automobile with Soy (2007, July 26). Retrieved August 20, 2007, from Web site: http://unitedsoybean.org

CHAPTER 7

Health Claims

I wrote in the beginning that I'd be fair, and that's what I'll do as I try to make sense of some of the research claims. Don't expect that kind of fairness from the soy industry. They report good news about soy, and they play down the questionable issues. I want you to at least be aware of both sides.

So, is soy a great food or a dangerous poison?

Let's examine some of the so called benefits. Is soy good for your heart? The FDA "consumers branch" thought so in 1999, but the FDA scientists disagreed. It approved wording for packaging claims that "diets low in saturated fat and cholesterol" with 25 grams of soy protein a day "may reduce the risk of heart disease."[1] The American Heart Association also supported soy as a heart helper. However, research during the next five years told a different story. The AHA withdrew its support for soy and soy supplements in 2005,[2] and the FDA may be ready to take another look at the research.[3]

The American Heart Association advisory panel reviewed 22 studies and found that an average of 50 grams of "isolated soy protein with isoflavones" mostly didn't reduce cholesterol or at best reduced it by a modest 3 percent. "This reduction is very small relative to the large amount of soy protein tested in these studies."[4]

How would you know something like that? You are more likely to see "Eat More Soy Protein, Lower Cholesterol," which is the heading of a 2006 article on the Tulane University Web site.[5] The article says that a Tulane researcher reviewed 41 studies and concluded that soy *can* reduce cholesterol. But when you read the whole article it's not what the Tulane researcher found. The research actually concluded, "Replacing foods high in saturated fat, trans-saturated fat and cholesterol with soy foods, such as tofu or soy milk, should be beneficial to cardiovascular health." Doesn't it sound like eating healthy foods should be beneficial to cardiovascular health?

And that's how Reuters reported the Tulane research, stating that the effect of soy in most of the 41 studies was too slight to prove anything.[6] Reuters reported the Tulane researcher herself as saying the key is not soy, but replacing foods that are high in saturated fats or cholesterol. The study doesn't actually show that soy protein as such has anything to do with lowering cholesterol.

This lack of clarity from many studies doesn't stop the soy industry's cheerleaders. In 2006, the Soy Daily Club Web site published an editorial that claims soy has many benefits, "including multiple studies that have *proven* that consumption of foods containing soy protein can play a *significant* role in cholesterol management [my italics]."[7]

Is it really proven or significant? It's clearly not proven, and even the most positive of the 41 research studies shows only a small decrease in cholesterol. Doesn't it make more sense to just skip the "magic soy formula" and spend your shopping dollars on fruits, vegetables, meats, and other healthy food?

Now we'll examine the isoflavones that the industry often touts as beneficial. First, according to *Endocrinology*, isoflavones are chemicals found in plants, and some of them have estrogen-like effects on the body.[8] These kinds of isoflavones are called phytoestrogens, and the two that are often written about are genistein and daidzein. Soybeans contain relatively large amounts of these two phytoestrogens. Information from the Soy Daily Club and a variety of other industry sources on a 2005 Snack and Bakery Web page states, "Current research suggests that soy may lower the risk of colon, prostate and breast cancers in addition to lowering the risk for high blood pressure and osteoporosis, and giving menopausal women relief from their symptoms."[9] Statements like this would make anyone a believer!

Another article from iHerb site says. "According to some but not all studies, soy protein or concentrated isoflavones from soy...may reduce menopausal symptoms such as hot flashes and vaginal dryness." Great! "Isoflavones decrease the action of regular estrogen by blocking estrogen receptor sites, and may also reduce levels of circulating estrogen. Since estrogen promotes breast and uterine cancer, these effects could help prevent breast cancer." Sounds good, but "only a large, long-term intervention trial could actually show that soy or isoflavones reduce breast and uterine cancer risk, and one has not been performed."[10]

You see, carefully worded reporting in scientific research doesn't support these heath claims. But, what if "may reduce" turns out to be "does reduce"? We're talking about powerful chemical agents. It reminds me of when penicillin was discovered by accident from bread mold. But wait until science figures out what's going on before you start eating moldy bread!

There's plenty of carefully worded research that questions all of these claims. The AHA advisory panel report of 2006 completely retracted claims about soy and heart health and stated that neither soy nor isoflavones have been shown to lesson the effects of menopause and that the results are at best mixed about bone loss. The advisory panel went on to say that the supposed benefits of soy on breast and prostate cancer are not established.[11]

So how can the soy industry continue to claim that soy lowers the risk of colon, prostate, and breast cancers? And, how can the industry still claim that soy lowers the risk for high blood pressure and osteoporosis, and that it is effective against hot flashes?

> *"I have always been a relatively healthy woman. Now at 48 years old, I've been taking "Revival" products for about 3 years and recently began eating soy nuts. Although my TSH levels were normal, my sonogram found multiple goiters that I need to see an endocrinologist about. After reading many testimonials about soy effects, I've decided to completely stop consuming products with soy. I hope I will not need surgery."*

In 2005, the FDA gave a number of Web sites 15 days to stop making unfounded health claims about soy, including one site that claimed soy can prevent cancer at multiple sites and inhibit the growth of cancerous cells. Also, that soy extract could be used in place of Premarin in hormone replacement therapy.[12] However, just put "Soy health benefits" (without the quotation marks) into your favorite Internet search engine and see what you get. I got two-and-a-half million hits! Some of them question the benefits, but most tout soy in the same way as the Web sites that the FDA busted.

Other than the questionable claims about the benefits, are there other reasons to be cautious about the phytoestrogens in soy? How about a 2000 study that concluded that genistein is an "endocrine disrupter" and that it increases one kind of breast cancer in rats?[13] Okay, so phytoestrogens like genistein and diadzein are endocrine disruptors. Isn't that what's supposed to be good about them, that they can interrupt estrogen and help prevent breast cancer and osteoporosis? What's this about increasing one kind of breast cancer? That's what science is still working on: how phytoestrogens work with estrogen, how much is too much, and, especially, when is the right time to disrupt the endocrine system. Science can't answer a single one of those questions right now. If you are eating soy products, you are part of a huge uncontrolled experiment. You are one of millions of two-legged lab rats.

"Two years ago I was diagnosed with hypothyroidism *due to excessive weight gain, hair falling out by the hands full, aches and pains and PVC's. Two months before attaining these symptoms, I began a regiment of one Estroven tablet daily due to low estrogen levels. I had never had a problem with taking the Estroven. It is fortunate that for whatever reason I stopped taking it when I was diagnosed. I will forever be on medication and deal with symptoms coming and going due to false advertisement. Thank you for sharing your website. I am hoping this reaches women in time before they have to suffer like many of us have already.*"

I know it's troubling to hear that we are the guinea pigs, but until we raise our voices and not wait for them to decide what experiments need to be done, nothing will change—especially because of the huge profits this industry is making.

So, you say, "I can make my own decisions about what to eat." Well what about your unborn child or your infant? Even though the scientists are using mice and rats—not people—research is raising red flags that you need to know about.

A 2005 genistein study on mice from birth until they were sexually mature "indicates that there are problems with female reproductive development and function."[14] The mice were not able to carry pups to term or were not able to deliver live pups. The researchers felt, as I do, that it was important to be aware of human implications. But in particular, "Infants exposed to high levels of phytoestrogens...such as Gen [genistein] in soy-based infant formulas and other soy products are of most concern."[15] A study published in the Lancet in 1997 found, "The daily exposure of infants to isoflavones in soy infant-formulas is 6-11 fold higher on a bodyweight basis than the dose that has hormonal effects in adults consuming soy foods."[16] Instead of uncritically believing the hype from the soy industry, I'm going to stick with science: "Additional studies are warranted on infants who are exposed to high levels of GEN [genistein] during development before concluding that such exposure is safe."[17]

I received the following:

> *"When I was pregnant, eating soy was followed by pain in my breasts. I researched soy and discovered it is high in estrogen. I have avoided it since then, but I notice that if I eat soy accidentally, my nursing son gets breasts."*

Is there something we need to do in light of these infant health issues? We could wait and let scientists take the lead. Growing numbers of scientists have done just that in several countries—the U.S., Canada, Britain, and New Zealand.[18,19,20,21]But I hope you will not wait for the slow pace of scientists and government agencies to begin cautioning the public. I hope we can make our doubts heard through petitions and blogs. In fact, though, scientists are being heard. The governments of Britain and New Zealand have issued official guidelines recommending that parents use soy infant formulas only when recommended by their pediatrician[22]; for example, when a baby can't tolerate breast milk or cow's milk. Parents choose soy formula because they believe that it is less allergenic than cow's milk even though soybeans themselves are a major allergen, but highly processed unfermented products loaded with phytates, enzyme inhibitors, rancid fatty acids and altered protein most certainly are not easy to digest.

The claim is that soy is an acceptable substitute for milk in the feeding of babies and young children. The main ingredient of soy-based infant formula is soy protein isolate, so along with the growth-depressing trypsin inhibitors, these formulas have a high phytate content. The use of soy formula has caused zinc deficiency in infants that is important to the development of the nervous system. Aluminum content of soy formula is ten times greater than that of milk-based formula and has a toxic effect on the kidneys of infants. Soy formulas lack cholesterol, which is essential for the development of the brain and the nervous system. Mothers' milk has a special enzyme that helps the baby absorb cholesterol. Cholesterol is also very important for the development and the integrity of the intestinal wall. Formulas are made with sucrose rather than lactose and galactose, which are human milk sugars that play an important role in the development of the nervous system. Soy formulas used to have lactose added, but that was too expensive, so now they just add sucrose. Not surprisingly, animal-feeding studies show a lower weight gain for rats on soy formula than for those on whole milk, high lactose formula.[23]

> *"My little girl is in trouble. She's just short of 2 years and hasn't grown or added any weight since April. According to her charts, she's had a regular growth and weight pattern that suddenly flat lined. Over these past five months her caloric intake through solid foods have dropped. She drinks six - 4 oz. bottles of Silk Soy Milk a day. We'll that was until tonight. About three weeks ago my wife and I had a number of blood tests performed on her. For the most part, the results have come back fine - with one exception - a blood test revealed that she's dehydrated - possible kidney issues. We are waiting a urinary test result and another blood test taken earlier today. My gut says, and her growth chart graph shows, that everything shifted the day we switched her to Soy. She's full of energy, very aware, speaks-using full sentences, and seems perfectly normal. She's just small and has not grown beyond April."*

Some of soy's hormonal effects may be reversible in adults following restoration of normal estrogen activity, but in newborns, the effects are more likely to be irreversible.[24]

I am not "cherry picking" the research to make a point. You can use the same words on an Internet search engine and find many articles that raise these same issues. These aren't scientists with an axe to grind with the soy industry. They are just making disturbing discoveries and reporting them. They are the same scientists who also investigate possible positive effects of soy. There may be potential for pharmaceutical drugs. But potential won't repair any long-term developmental damage to children.

You will read some real horror stories in Chapter 12.

"My daughter is 15 months old and she has breast budding. The pediatrician ordered an estradiol test that revealed abnormal amounts of estrogen in her body. Normal ranging from 5-10 and my daughters were at a 23. I decided to stop her consumption of soymilk, and BEHOLD in 2 wks, her estradiol test revealed an 8, which is perfectly normal. My pediatrician is now completing documentation on this soy issue. I am grateful that this was detected early. I fear she may have had severe side effects such as precocious puberty, thyroid, etc. I want to do everything possible to prevent this from happening to another child before it is too late! I plan on creating a website and writing to baby magazines in hopes that it will prevent parents from going through the emotional roller coaster I was riding prior to her normal test results. Initially, I was told that my daughter may have a mass in the brain that could be producing estrogen, however, it was soy. I am grateful that is was soy, but I am also disturbed that soy is still on the market."

While the industry is quick to use words like *proven* and *significant* when touting soy, they are just as quick to use *unproven* when talking about the dangers. "American Institute for Cancer Research stresses that data on soy and breast cancer is not conclusive."[25] Earlier we established "Compounds that bind to estrogen receptors often have different, and sometimes opposite, physiological effects depending upon how the isoflavone and receptor interact within different cells."[26] Yes, that's what the scientists figured. I know it's complicated because it's not easy for me to understand either.

The industry wants to play down the research by pointing out it's done in a lab, not in real life, but considering how my health improved since I had to remove soy from my diet, and all the testimonials you will read, this is proof enough for me!

"I am a 30-year-old vegetarian who has been taking in around 40-50 grams of soy protein a day. I have recently started having problems with heart palpitations and weight gain. I am on the Weight Watchers points system and I have gained 11 lb. in 2 1/2 months. I have been very disturbed by this gain, knowing that I am exercising 5-6 days a week and staying very active every day. Everyone else on WW is losing except for me it seems. My grandmother was diagnosed with thyroid disease many years ago and I seem to have all the symptoms such as, weight gain, palpitations, memory loss. I read articles that made me aware that soy is to blame. I don't know if I have already damaged my thyroid, but I am going to stop my soy intake today!"

Let's give the parting words about soy isoflavones to an FDA magazine article: "While isoflavones may have beneficial effects at some ages or circumstances, this cannot be assumed to be true at all ages. Isoflavones are like other estrogens are two-edged swords, conferring both benefits and risks." And, "Research data, however, are far from conclusive...It is this scientific conundrum, where evidence simultaneously points to benefits and possible risks, that is causing some researchers to urge caution."[27]

If the FDA and other researchers are urging caution, don't you think you should too? We're talking about your long-term health.

[1] Food and Drug Administration. (1999, October 20). FDA approves new health claim for soy protein and coronary heart disease. *Federal Talk Paper*. Retrieved May 29, 2007, from http://www.cfsan.fda.gov/~lrd/tpsoypr2.html

[2] American Heart Association. (2006, January 17). Soy protein, isoflavones, and cardiovascular health. *Circulation, 113*, 1034-1044. Retrieved July 11, 2007, from http://circ.ahajournals.org/cgi/content/abstract/CIRCULATIONAHA.106.171052v1

[3] Boyles, S. (2006, January 23). Soy heart benefits questioned. *WebMD Medical News*. Retrieved June 28, 2007, from http://www.webmd.com/news/20060123/soys-heart-benefits-questioned

[4] American Heart Association

[5] Nead, A. (2006, September 29). Eat more soy protein, lower cholesterol. Retrieved July 7, 2007, from Tulane University Web site: http://www2.tulane.edu/article_news_details.cfm?ArticleID=6827

[6] China Daily. (2006, September 22). Soy protein lowers cholesterol slightly. *Reuters*. Retrieved July 11, 2007, from http://www.chinadaily.com.cn/world/2006-09/22/content_694737.htm

[7] Gieseke, T. (2006). Soy foods becoming synonymous with health & wellness. Retrieved June 26, 2007, from Soy Daily Club Web site: http://thesoydailyclub.com/DisplayEditorial.cfm?EditorialID=2
I have a copy of this editorial, but the URL no longer works, and I can't find it in the Soy Daily Club archives.

[8] Patisaul, H. B., Dindo, M., Whitten, P. L., & Young, L. J. (2001). Soy isoflavone supplements antagonize reproductive behavior and estrogen receptor α- and ß-dependent gene expression in the brain. *Endocrinology, 142*(7), 2946-2952. Retrieved June 10, 2007, from http://endo.endojournals.org/cgi/content/full/142/7/2946

[9] Clark, M. P. (2007). Soy luck club. Retrieved July 7, 2007, from Snack Food & Wholesale Bakery Web site: http://www.snackandbakery.com/content.php?s=SF/2005/02&p=22

[10] iHerb (n.d.) Isoflavones. Retrieved July 11, 2007, from iHerb Web site: http://healthlibrary.epnet.com/GetContent.aspx?token=e0498803-7f62-4563-8d47-5fe33da65dd4&chunkiid=21778

[11] American Heart Association

[12] Baca, J. R. (2005, November 9). Food and Drug Administration Warning Letter. Retrieved April 13, 2007, from
http://www.casewatch.org/fdawarning/prod/2005/estrofemme.shtml

[13] Yang, J., Nakagawa, H., Tsuta, K., & Tsubura, A. (2000, February 28). Influence of perinatal genistein exposure on the development of MNU-induced mammary carcinoma in female Sprague-Dawley rats. Cancer Letter, *149*(1-2), 171-179. Retrieved June 11, 2007, from
http://www.medscape.com/medline/abstract/10737721

[14] Jefferson, W. N., Patilla-Banks, E., & Newbold, R. R. (2005, June 1). Adverse effects on female development and reproduction in CD-1 mice following neonatal exposure to the phytoestrogen genistein at environmentally relevant doses. *Biology Of Reproduction, 73*, 798–806. Retrieved June 10, 2007, from
http://www.biolreprod.org/cgi/content/full/73/4/798

[15] Jefferson, W. N., Patilla-Banks, E., & Newbold, R. R.

[16] Setchell, K. D., Zimmer-Nechemias. L., Cai, J., & Heubi, J. E. (1997, July 5). Exposure of infants to phyto-oestrogens from soy-based infant formula. *Lancet, 350*(9070), 23-27. Abstract retrieved July 21, 2007, from
http://www.ncbi.nlm.nih.gov/sites/entrez?cmd=retrieve&db=pubmed&list_uids=9217716&dopt=Abstract

[17] Jefferson, W. N., Patilla-Banks, E., & Newbold, R. R.

[18] Nutra Ingredients News (2003, May 2). Soy formula needs to be reviewed, say UK scientists. Retrieved August 3, 2007, from Web site:
http://nutraingredients.com/news/news-NG.asp?n=37795-soy-formula-needs

[19] Henkel, J. (2000, May-June). Soy: Health claims for soy protein, questions about other components. *FDA Consumer, 34*(3). Retrieved June 28, 2007, from
http://www.fda.gov/fdac/features/2000/300_soy.html

[20] Natural Life Magazine. (1999, July-August). Soy infant formula dangerous to babies, say groups. Retrieved August 3, 2007, from Web site:
http://www.life.ca/nl/68/formula.html

[21] New Zealand Food Safety Authority. (2003). Soy-based infant formula. Retrieved August 3, 2007, from http://www.nzfsa.govt.nz/consumers/food-safety-topics/chemicals-in-food/soy-infant-milk-formula/index.htm

[22] New Zealand Food Safety Authority.

[23] Fallon, S., http://www.consumerhealth.org. Retreived June 7, 2007

[24] Daniel, K.T., The Whole Soy Story, the dark side of America's health food, New Trends Publishing , Inc. 2005 (p.333)

[25] Tsang, G. (2006, February). Powerful benefits of soy. Retrieved June 28, 2007, from Healthcastle Nutrition, Inc., Web site:
http://www.healthcastle.com/herb_soy.shtml

[26] Soy Nutrition (n.d.). Myths about soy. Retrieved June 28, 2007, from Soy Nutrition Web site: http://www.soynutrition.com/SoyHealth/SoyMyths.aspx

[27] Henkel, J.

CHAPTER 8

Should You Avoid Soy?

I gave you plenty to think about in the last chapter. There is evidence that soy may contain chemicals that can help us in the future, but there is evidence that soy is hurting us right now. In this chapter, I want to give you my opinion on soy products. You may be saying to yourself, "Well, she has a severe allergy to soy, and I don't!" That is true, but I wouldn't eat soy products now even if I didn't have the allergy. I know too much now.

Even though there are claims that suggest modest amounts of soy are safe, do you know how much soy you're getting? I believe you'll be surprised when you read Chapter 9 on Where the Soy is Hidden. You're getting more than you think.

Here are some of the very serious issues that people have been raising for years. Research is just scratching the surface about whether the dangers are real or not, but I don't want my future generations to suffer.

Promoters of soy products such as soy protein isolate, or phyto-estrogens extracted from soy, usually fail to mention that soy products are goitrogenic to humans. That means they depress thyroid function. Certain substances found in the soybean inhibit thyroid hormone synthesis, leading to goiter and other adverse changes in the thyroid gland. Low thyroid function is associated with a host of debilitating diseases including cancer, heart disease, fatigue, osteoporosis, and a difficult menopause. So, if you are taking soy for your menopause, it is depressing your thyroid and it may cause you to have a more difficult menopause. Try eating whole nutrient dense foods including animal fats, but avoid processed commercial foods.[1]

Isoflavones can inhibit thyroid peroxidase (TPO), an enzyme involved in the synthesis of thyroid hormones.[2] As their name implies, some research suggests that goitrogens can cause an enlarged thyroid, known as a *goiter*, by increasing the amount of thyroid stimulating hormone. People can get goiters and other thyroid problems from either an iodine deficiency or in some cases from iodine excess. Iodine is important in other areas of metabolic regulation.[3]

I just wanted to add here that Christiane Northrup, MD, author of The Wisdom of Menopause, is a big promoter of soy, and did you know she has hypothyroidism? What a coincidence!

If you are menopausal and gaining weight, did it ever occur to you that you could be developing a thyroid problem?

The claim that soy foods prevent cancer is predicated on two suppositions: 1) that Asian populations consume large amounts of soy foods; 2) that Asian populations have low amounts of cancer. The average consumption in China is 9 gm - that is less than a tablespoon, and the average consumption in Japan is 30 gm, which is between two and three tablespoons. Yet, *The Simple Soy Bean and Your Health* recommends one cup, or 230 grams of soy products per day in an optimal diet to prevent cancer. This amount is not consumed in the Orient. And, these are the traditional soy products being consumed, not the soy protein isolate. Studies have shown that consumption of legumes is not strongly correlated with the prevention of any degenerative disease, including cancer. Some studies, in fact, link the actual consumption of soy foods with increased rates of cancer. Why are rates of breast cancer astronomically high in the U.S.? It's because of the consumption of soy foods in the form of *hydrogenated margarines and shortenings.* These trans-fats in our food supply contribute to breast cancer. With so many books on the market on how to prevent breast cancer, none of them even mention the very carcinogenic effects on breast tissue of these trans-fatty acids.[4]

If I had breast cancer or was at high risk for breast cancer, I would definitely eliminate soy until more is known. Look at all the women that stopped taking HRT because of the risks? In a newsletter by The Gerson Insitute, Dr. Max Gerson has soy on the "forbidden" list for his cancer patients.[5] What does this tell you?

Of course, some people are allergic to soy and should avoid it (duh!). Other people say they feel better when not eating soy. And other people feel better when they do eat soy. I've been told by nutrionists that people who feel better taking soy (euphoria) is only temporary because there is so much sugar in it to camaflouge the awful taste of the soybean that your body gets use to it and then the euphoria fades. That's when the tables can turn and you start feeling lousy, which could indicate a problem is starting to develop. So, you never know. So how safe is it?

I received the following testionial from my website:

> *I am a celiac (wheat allergy) who is also very allergic to soy and I'm appalled that it is used in everything! I have long been convinced that soy is responsible for premature puberty, obesity, and other problems. I've also made it my mission to tell people of the dangers. Thank you!*

According to SoyOnlineService, soy formulas are over-supplemented with minerals and vitamins to account for the deficiencies caused by phytate, but this does not take care of the problems. The removal of phytate from soy formulas would be a better solution. But the manufactures have not been willing to do it. This point is frustrating when manufacturers consider profits more important than the well being of infants. [6]

The French Food Agency will soon require warning labels on all soy foods, soy formulas and soy milk so that consumers will be aware of the risks that soy poses to children under the age of three, as well as people with hypothyroidism, and women with a family history of breast cancer.[7]

Well, how about this testmonial?

> *"As the mother of a 4-year-old boy, I'd like to add my 2 cents regarding the extreme health hazards of soy. My son was born with a 3rd degree hypospadias, which required 10 surgeries to correct. He had the worst hypospadias a male can have, where his urethra's opening appeared at the base of his genitals. How did this utter nightmare occur? Well, little did I know that the DAILY tofu and soymilk I was drinking for the past decade (I was foolishly a vegan) was highly estrogenating my already estrogenated body. Healthy women make enough estrogen as it is. The phytoestrogens disrupted my fetus' development. I have met other women who had sons with hypospadias and they ate soy daily all during pregnancy.*
>
> *Enough said. Thank you for helping the public realize how detrimental soy is, and that it's really just junk food."*

An issue that we may hear more about as research

accumulates is the possibility that soy foods may be part of the skyrocketing diagnoses of behavior problems in children. I'm not trying to "pile on" by saying that soy is the cause of so many different kinds of problems, but you need to be aware of the possibility. According to the *New York Times*, bipolar diagnoses increase by 4000 percent between 1994 and 2003 for children and adolescents.[8] Part of the increase is without doubt caused by the condition receiving more attention, but a 40-fold increase can't be explained away.

The *Times* article went on to say that most of the children had "other mental difficulties, mostly attention deficit disorder." A study in 2002 at the University of California-Irvine "discovered that a mineral found in high levels in soy milk appears to be linked to behavioral problems. The study in rats, one of the first scientific inquiries into soy milk and ADHD, indicates that the mineral manganese may cause behavioral problems if consumed in high doses."[9] The study showed that soymilk contains 80 times the amount of manganese as breast milk does. And rats fed with high doses had lower levels of dopamine, and they had problems with completing tasks.

> *"I have a 15 year old daughter who fits the description of a soy fed infant. She was fed soy formula for almost 2 years because she did not tolerate milk. I think she has hormone imbalances that are causing various problems physically and emotionally. My daughter has abnormally excess body hair. This is not specifically mentioned as a symptom. From what I understood from the articles I have read about this excess hair condition and the soy, the ovaries are "in charge" of stimulating androgens and testosterone hormones. Testosterone is the hormone that stimulates*

> *hair growth. My daughter began having pubic hair around the age of 5 and I remember noticing a swollen look to her as an infant when I changed her diaper. It always concerned me, but I could never connect a cause. These conditions are not specifically mentioned as symptoms of the soy, but I speculate it is related. She also has asthma, allergies, ADHD, started gaining weight last year without reason, (no diet has been successful) and has irregular menstrual cycles."*

In August 2007, I interviewed a 51-year-old man who was a vegetarian since the age of 25 and ate lots of soy. By the time he was 45 years old, he weighed 230lbs. One morning when he awoke, he wasn't feeling well. He couldn't stop throwing up and passed out momentarily. He stayed in bed the rest of the day. The next morning, he had double vision, and a loss of balance. At that point, he evaluated his diet and realized he had tofu 3 days in a row. A month later, he was feeling better but decided to see the doctor. At this point, he now weighed 240lbs. The doctor checked his blood pressure 275/168 and told him he couldn't believe he is still alive – what happened was he had a stroke! After reading, *"The Whole Soy Story"* by Dr. Kaayla Daniel, he realized that soy was contributing to his illnesses. He is still a vegetarian, but he took soy completely out of his diet. He went back to his normal weight of 185 within months. Two years ago, he started a soy free restaurant and cooks everything from scratch!

The following testimonials I found from the Gerson Institute Newsletter Volume 14 #3:

> *November/December: A pregnant woman who looked very ill, was also terribly deficient! She also described her son, age five, who had many allergies and infections – both*

were using a good deal of soy in their diet. I recommended that they discontinue the use of all soy products. At the time, I had only just run across this situation. However, a year later, I was in the same area for a lecture, and the lady invited me to dinner. She had cut out all soy products: her skin was now rosy, her face filled out, her sunken eyes normal, her black circles gone and her little boy, now six, was in greatly improved health.

November 1998: "I have used soy milk for 12 years with no problems. About 9 months ago, I started to have heart palpitations. I thought maybe that I was in menopause, but I wasn't. I added more potassium to my diet and magnesium and vitamin E. No change. I am already decaffeinated but I also took all sugar out of my diet. I lost 25 pounds and felt great except for the palpitations. I tried hawthorn and garlic but nothing was helping. Recently I came down with acute bronchitis and could only drink water because even the soymilk made me have horrendous bouts of coughing. I realized that after a few days my heart palpitations had stopped. I didn't think anything of it because it never occurred to me that soy was the culprit. As soon as I started drinking it again, my heart went crazy. I went off it for a week and then changed brands. Within 30 minutes of drinking only 4 ounces of soymilk, my heart was all over the place. I've noticed that it takes about 24 to 36 hours for my heart to settle down."

A patient at the Gerson Certified Hospital in Mexico told us of her son, now 25, has total lack of hair (Alopecia) with the exception of eyebrows and eyelashes. She said this started when he was just three years old. Since the mother asked me about this situation, I considered the problem for a moment. After looking at the parents who both have normal hair, I figured the boy's problem was not genetic. I asked the mother if he used a lot of soy. She said, no. But then, remembered that at about one year of

---

age, the boy had many allergies, so she regularly fed him soymilk! I explained to her that the enzyme and nutrient blocking ability of soy and the likelihood of the soy milk being the cause of his condition starting at age three. Since we had just witnessed the case of a patient whose hair grew back on his baldpate, after being bald for some 20 years, I cautiously suggested that a complete change of diet with intensive detoxification, might be able to overcome the problem.

I will end this chapter by letting you decide for yourself. I hope you will consider the researchers' warnings.

[1] Fallon, S., http://www.consumerhealth.org, Retrieved June 7, 2007

[2] Duncan, A. M., & Dillingham, B. L. (2006, Summer). Soy & thyroid function: Safety issues examined. *The Soy Connection, 14*(3), 1-3. Retrieved April 14, 2007, from: http://www.soyconnection.com/upload/SCNv14n3.pdf

[3] Duncan, A. M., & Dillingham, B. L. (2006, Summer). Soy & thyroid function: Safety issues examined. *The Soy Connection, 14*(3), 1-3. Retrieved April 14, 2007, from: http://www.soyconnection.com/upload/SCNv14n3.pdf

[4] Fallon, S., Enig Mary G, Nourishing Traditions, New Trends Publishing, Inc. 2nd Edition 2001

[5] Finucan, B., & Gerson, C., (2000, February 13). Soy: Too good to be true. *Gerson Institute Newsletter,14*(3). Retrieved April 5, 2007, from http://www.becomehealthynow.com/article/soy/1085

[6] SoyOnlineService (n.d.) Soy toxins. Retrieved May 10, 2007, from Web site: http://www.soyonlineservice.co.nz/03toxins.htm

[7] http://www.AllergyKids.com

[8] Carey, B. (2007, September 4). Bipolar Illness soars as a diagnosis for the young. *New York Times.*

9 Is there a link (2002, October 7). Is there a link between soy formula and attention deficit disorder? Scientific study of soymilk finds behavior problems from high manganese levels. Science *Daily*

CHAPTER 9

Where The Soy Is Hidden

W e are eating soy products today at levels never before seen in history. Advances in food technology have made it possible to isolate soy proteins, isoflavones, and other substances found in the bean and add them to all kinds of foods where they've never been before. The number of processed and manufactured foods that contain soy ingredients today is astounding. As I have mentioned before, it can be hard to find foods that don't contain soy flour, soy oil, lecithin (extracted from soy oil and used as an emulsifier in high-fat products), soy protein isolates and concentrates, textured vegetable protein (TVP), hydrolyzed vegetable protein (usually made from soy) or unidentified vegetable oils. Most of what is labeled "vegetable oil" in the U.S. is actually soy oil, as are most margarines. Soy oil is the most widely used oil in the U.S., accounting for more than 75 percent of our total vegetable fats and oil intake. And most of our soy products are now genetically engineered. This is where my frustration comes in because of my limitations when purchasing food from the grocery store.

The following ingredients I retrieved from Web Site http://www.mercola.com will help you know what to look for on the labels.

Obviously, the first section (common names of soy products) is easy to identify.

I bet when you read the rest of this list you will be astonished as to how many ingredients have soy that you were not aware of. That's why it is so important to read the labels. And, why it's impossible to only eat 2-3 servings of soy a day.

Now you can understand why someone like me with a severe allergy to soy needs to be very careful and get creative with my cooking.

As always, use extra precaution when eating out at restaurants or eating foods prepared by others if you suspect you have an allergy.

Common names of soy products / Always contains it:

Edamame
Miso – consumed in moderation – fermentation not proper or adequate
Natto – consumed in moderation – fermentation not proper or adequate
Shoyu
Tamari
Tempeh – consumed in moderation – fermentation not proper or adequate
Texturized vegetable protein (TVP)
Tofu – not so good as you would expect
Soymilk
Soy sauce
Soy nuts
Soy grits
Soy protein
Soy protein isolate
Soybean paste / curd
Miso
Sobee
Kyodofu (freeze-dried tofu)
Soy sprouts
Soy flour
Soy/tofu cheese
Soy yogurt

These ingredients may contain soy if the source has not been specified:

Bulking agent
Emulsifier
Guar gum
Gum Arabic
Hydrolyzed vegetable protein (HVP)
Hydrolyzed plant protein (HPP)
Lecithin
Protein filler/extender
Mono-& diglycerides
MSG (monosodium glutamate)
Seasoned salt
Shortenings
Stabilizer
Thickener
Vegetable/gum/starch/oil/protein

Common Sources / Foods Containing Soy

Baby food
Canned fish
Chocolates (creamed centers)
Cooking oils
High protein bars/ foods
Ice cream/frozen desserts
Dessert mixes
Margarine
Mayonnaise
Meat products
Powdered meal replacers
Baked goods
Breakfast cereals (mixed grain/multi grain)
Infant cereals
High protein flour and bread

Stuffings
Mixed sprouts
Salad sprouts
Salad dressings
Canned soup/dried soup mixes
Vegetarian meat replacers
Frozen dinners
Mixed bean preparation
Prepared sauces, e.g. Barbecue, oriental, etc.
Chocolate
Sauces (Asian, gravy, soy, Worcestershire)
Shortening

CHAPTER 10

Soy-Free Recipes

Chicken Soup
6 - 8 Servings

1-32oz Container of Kitchen Basics Chicken Stock
2 cups of water
2 medium onions sliced
6 carrots cut
3 stalks of celery cut
1Tbsp dill
1 tsp white vinegar
Salt and Pepper to taste
1 Whole chicken cut-up – I remove the skin

Add the first eight ingredients, bring to boil, and then add cut-up chicken
Stir all ingredients, cover pot, and simmer for 2-3 hours.

*Vinegar helps draw out the bone marrow from the chicken bones making this soup healthier. Use the vinegar when making beef stock as well. Substitute beef bones.

Italian Minnestrone Soup
4 Servings

2 8oz cans dark red kidney beans, drained
2 32oz Kitchen Basic Beef Stock
3-4 cloves garlic, minced
3 Tbsp olive oil
1 Lg. yellow onion, chopped
3 Lg. carrots, sliced
3 celery stalks sliced
1 Lg. white potato, diced
1 8 oz.can peeled diced tomatoes
1 8oz. can corn
1 Medium size zucchini
1 cup small ditalini (follow cooking directions on package)
Salt and pepper
1 Tbsp Oregano
1 Tbsp Basil
½ cup grated Parmesan cheese

Combine beef stock, salt & pepper, oregano and basil. Bring to a boil. Add kidney beans, lower heat to simmer.

Sauté carrots, onions, garlic, celery, zucchini, and potato in heated olive oil until well coated with oil.

Add to beef stock bringing to a boil again, then turn to low. Cover and simmer for 30 – 40 minutes.

Add diced tomatoes, corn, and pre-cooked ditalini.

Sweet N' Sour Chicken
4 - 6 Servings

1 Whole Chicken cut-up, Skinless Chicken Breast,
Thighs, or drumsticks can be used.
½ cup Apricot Preserve
½ cup Orange Marmalade
1 cup orange juice – not from concentrate
1 Tbsp Honey

Season Chicken with salt and pepper. Sprinkle with
garlic powder and onion powder. And paprika, on both
sides.

Place chicken in a casserole dish. Mix the orange juice
in the marmalade and the preserves with the honey.
Spoon it on top of chicken leaving about a ¼ cup for
reserve. Add water to bottom of casserole dish.

Bake at 350 degrees – basting occasionally to keep the
chicken moist until done approximately 45 minutes.

Spoon remaining ¼ cup of the preserves before
serving. Serve with rice and a vegetable (when making
the rice, substitute the chicken stock instead of water
to add extra flavor, or add some remaining preserves).

Rolled Swiss Chicken Cutlets
4 Servings

Two slices Swiss cheese
4 Chicken cutlets (4oz each – ¼" thick) (You can buy 2
boneless chicken breasts, and pound to ¼" thickness,
then cut each breast lengthwise to make 4)
2 Tbs all-purpose flour & ½ tsp black pepper mixed
together
1 Tbs Butter (or olive oil)
½ cup chicken broth
½ cup dry white wine (optional) or ½ broth
¼ tsp oregano

Cut each cheese slice in half and place on top of each
cutlet. Tightly roll up cutlets and secure with string.

Toss chicken rolls gently in flour & pepper mixture

In large skillet, melt butter over medium heat. Add
cutlets, turning frequently, until golden brown (about
3 minutes).

Add broth, wine and oregano to skillet. Increase heat
bringing to a boil. Reduce heat to medium-low;
simmer until chicken is cooked and sauce is slightly
thickened, about 10-12 minutes.

Serve on white, brown or wild rice.

Easy Garlic-Stuffed Chicken
4 Servings

4 Boneless chicken breasts with skin
8 tsp chopped garlic
6 Tbsp dried parsley, divided
1 tsp grated lemon peel (optional)
¼ tsp salt
½ cup Kitchen Basic Chicken Stock
2 Tbsp lemon juice

In a small bowl, combine 4 tsp chopped garlic, 3 Tbsp parsley, lemon peel, and salt. Mix well.

Loosen skin from chicken breast and place 1 tsp of garlic mixture under skin of each breast.

Add ¼ cup chicken stock, at medium-high heat bring to boil, and add chicken skin-side down. Cook about 4-5 minutes until golden brown, then turn chicken.

Cover and cook until no longer pink in center, about 10-12 minutes. Transfer chicken to plate.

Add remaining ingredients, bring to boil, about 1 minute. Spoon mixture over chicken.

Serve with white or wild rice, and steamed broccoli.

Chicken Salad
4-6 Servings

2 cooked chicken breasts
1 stalk of celery
1 slice onion chopped finely
1 McIntosh apple peeled, cored & chopped
Salt & Pepper to taste
¼ chopped walnuts
¼ cup raisins
¾ Hains Safflower or Canola Oil Mayonnaise

Chop chicken breasts in food Processor, and then add
remaining ingredients.
Serve on a salad or make sandwiches.

Tuna Fish Salad
2 Servings

1 8oz can StarKist Low Sodium Chunk Light Tuna in
Water (the only one without soy)
1 celery stalk diced
1/8 tsp of Lemon Pepper
1 slice onion chopped finely
¼ cup Hains Safflower or Canola Oil Mayonnaise

Mash tuna with fork and mix all ingredients together.

Serve on a salad with sliced cucumbers and green or
red pepper.
Or, soy free bread for sandwiches.

Sweet N' Sour Pork
4 Servings

4 Pork Loin Center Cut Pork Chops
4 Tbs flour
1 Tbs olive oil
½ cup Apricot Preserve
½ cup Orange Marmalade
1 cup orange juice – not from concentrate
1 Tbsp Honey

Bread pork chops with flour on both sides.

Preheat oven to 350 degrees.

In a large skillet heat olive oil, add pork chops until brown turning once.

Transfer pork chops to ovenproof casserole dish.

Mix the orange juice, marmalade, preserves, and honey. Spoon it on top of pork leaving about a ¼ cup for reserve. Add water to bottom of dish.

Bake at 350 degrees – basting occasionally to keep the pork moist until done approximately 20-30 minutes. Spoon the remaining ¼ cup of the preserves before serving.

Serve with rice and a vegetable (when making the rice, substitute the chicken stock instead of water to add extra flavor, or add some remaining preserves).

Shrimp and Spinach Pasta
4 Servings

8 oz. Angel hair pasta
1 tsp olive oil
1 tsp minced garlic
12 oz. Peeled, deveined medium-size fresh shrimp
¼ tsp dried crushed red pepper (optional)
1 (10oz.) bag pre-washed spinach leaves
2 plum tomatoes cut into eighths
2 Tbs fresh lemon juice
¼ tsp salt

Cook pasta according to package directions. Drain and reserve 3 tablespoons water.

While pasta cooks, add oil to skillet placing over medium-high heat until hot.

Add garlic, cook 1 minute stirring often. Add shrimp and red pepper, cook 2 minutes stirring often. Add spinach, tomato, lemon juice, salt and reserved pasta water; cover and cook 3 minutes or until spinach wilts and shrimp turns pink.

Combine all ingredients in a large bowl and toss gently.

Fillet of Sole in Mushroom Sauce
4 Servings

1Tbsp butter
2 Tbsp chopped shallots
4 fillets of sole
Salt & pepper to taste
1 cup dry white wine
½ cup coconut milk
2 Tbsp butter
1-1/2 cups sliced mushrooms

In a frying pan, melt butter and lightly sauté the shallots. Place the sole in the frying and season with salt & pepper. Add white wine, cover, and poach for 5 minutes. Do not overcook.

Remove fillets from pan and keep warm. Pour the coconut milk into frying pan and simmer for 2 minutes; add a little cornstarch to thicken while stirring. In another pan melt the 2 tbsp butter and lightly sauté mushrooms. Drain and add to the sauce. Pour mushroom sauce over the fish and serve with asparagus.

*You can substitute other fish for this recipe.

Shrimp Newburg
6 Servings

1 ½lb shrimp peeled & deveined
1/3-cup butter
½ cup flour
1-½ cups milk
1 Tbsp dry sherry or chicken stock
4 tsp fresh lemon juice
2 slices homemade soy-free French bread, cut into ½ inch cubes

Cook shrimp in boiling water 1-3 minutes or until opaque. Drain.

Preheat oven to 350 degrees. In medium saucepan melt ½ cup butter. Stir in flour and add milk stirring until thickened and bubbly. Stir in shrimp, lemon juice, and season to taste with salt and pepper.

Coat 2-quart baking dish with butter, and pour shrimp mixture into dish. Bake 15-20 minutes.

Stir together bread cubes and 1 Tbsp melted butter. Sprinkle over shrimp mixture. Bake 3-5 minutes more until topping is toasted.

*You can vary this recipe with crab, lobster, or scallops.
*Another variation would be to substitute bread with pasta without baking and pour mixture over pasta.

Shrimp Creole
6-8 Servings

2 pounds shrimp, rinsed, peeled and deveined
¼ cup butter
½ cup green bell pepper, diced ½"
½ cup onion, diced ¼"
¼ cup celery, chopped fine
1 clove garlic, minced
2 tablespoons flour, all purpose
1 can (14.5-oz) whole peeled tomatoes, roughly cut
1 teaspoon sugar
1 teaspoon salt
¼ teaspoon cayenne pepper
¼ teaspoon black pepper
4 cups cooked rice

In a small sauce pan, melt 2 tablespoons of butter over medium heat. Mix in flour and stir until dissolved and mixture begins to thicken, then reduce heat.

Add tomatoes and their juice to the butter and flour mixture, stir well, and heat through until the mixture thickens. Keep warm.

In a large skillet over medium high heat melt 2 tablespoons butter, cook bell pepper, onion, celery, and garlic until soft but with a little bit of a crunch.

Add shrimp and cook until no longer transparent (3 minutes). Add tomato mixture, bring to a boil, cover, and let simmer for 5 minutes. Serve over hot rice (white or wild).

Pecan-Crusted Tilapia
Serves 4

¾ cup chopped pecans
2 Tbsp cornmeal
2 Tbsp butter
4 Tilapia fillets

Preheat oven to 400 degrees. Coat baking dish with butter.

In blender or food processor pulse pecans and cornmeal until nuts are finely chopped.

Place fillets in baking dish, sprinkle with salt if desired, brush evenly with butter, and top with pecan mixture pressing lightly.

Bake for 12-18 minutes or until fish flakes easily.

Baked Salmon
2 Servings

2 Salmon Fillets (4-6oz each)
1 Tbs Lemon Pepper Seasoning
1 Tbs Honey
1 tsp orange juice

Preheat heat oven or toaster oven 350 degrees.

Bake or broil 6-8 minutes until pinkish, then
Combine honey and orange juice, then spoon over
salmon and cook another 2 minutes.

Serve with white or wild rice, and vegetable.

Roasted Vegetables
6-8 Servings

3 Red Bell Peppers
3 Yellow Bell Peppers
3 Orange Bell Peppers
2 onions sliced
1 Pkg Baby Bella mushrooms sliced
3 Yellow Squash sliced
2 Zucchinis sliced
1 Medium Eggplant peeled and cut in chunks
1cup olive oil
½ cup balsamic vinaigrette
1Tbsp honey.

In a skillet, add 1Tbsp olive oil and 1tsp butter. When heated add vegetables to sauté slightly. Place vegetables in a 13" x 9" dish sprinkle salt and pepper, thyme, basil, rosemary, tarragon, and a little dill, and oregano. Mix the last 3 ingredients together and pour onto vegetables, toss to cover all vegetables. Bake at 350 degrees for 30 minutes, tossing occasionally to evenly brown.

Roasted Asparagus with Pine Nuts
4 servings

2 Tbsp pine nuts
1 1/2 pounds asparagus
1 large shallot, thinly sliced
2 teaspoons extra-virgin olive oil
¼ tsp salt, divided
Freshly ground pepper to taste
¼ cup balsamic vinegar
1 tsp honey (optional)

Preheat oven to 350 degrees. Spread pine nuts in a small baking pan and toast in the oven until golden and fragrant, 7-10 minutes. Transfer to a small bowl to cool.

Increase oven temperature to 450 degrees.

Cut off the tough ends of asparagus. Toss the asparagus with shallot, oil, 1/8 tsp salt, and pepper. Spread in a single layer on a large baking sheet with sides. Roast for 5-7 minutes each side, until the asparagus are tender and browned.

Meanwhile, in a small skillet over medium-high heat, bring vinegar and remaining 1/8 teaspoon salt (add honey if desired) to a simmer. Reduce heat to medium-low and simmer, swirling the pan occasionally, until slightly syrupy and reduced to 1 tablespoon, about 5 minutes. To serve, toss the asparagus with the reduced vinegar and sprinkle with pine nuts.

Polynesian Pilaf
6 Servings

1 8oz. can pineapple tidbits in juice, drained (reserve juice)
2 cups uncooked instant white rice
2 cups snow peas
1 Tbsp. Packed brown sugar
2 tsp diced pimento
½ tsp ground ginger
½ tsp salt

In a 2 Quart saucepan, combine reserved pineapple juice and water to equal 1-2/3 cups.

Add remaining ingredients, except for pineapple.

Bring to boil, add rice, and stir. Cover and remove from heat. Let stand 5-7 minutes until rice is tender and liquid is absorbed.

Add pineapple, fluff rice with fork.

Garlic Mashed Potatoes
4 - 6 Servings

2 pounds red potatoes peeled or unpeeled (your choice)
8 Tbsp unsalted butter
½ cup milk
2 Tbsp minced garlic
Salt & Pepper to taste

Place potatoes cut in even chunks in large saucepan and bring to boil over high heat, then reduce heat and simmer until potatoes are tender 20-30 minutes. Drain. Place potatoes in food processor with butter, minced garlic, salt & pepper blend and gradually add milk. Blend on medium speed, scraping sides. Add more milk if you want mushier potatoes.

*Another variation would be to substitute garlic with 1 cup of grated Parmesan Cheese and 1/8 teaspoon of grated nutmeg.

Oven-Roasted Potatoes
2 Servings

2 medium baking potatoes
4 tablespoons olive oil
1/2 teaspoon salt
2 teaspoons fresh rosemary, chopped (or dried)
1 teaspoon fresh garlic, minced
4 teaspoons fresh parsley, chopped (or dried)
1/2 cup Romano cheese, grated

Preheat oven to 350 degrees F.

Peel potatoes and dice into1/2-inch pieces. Core and seed peppers and dice into1/2-inch pieces. Set aside.

Mix olive oil, rosemary, salt and pepper in a bow l.

In a small baking pan, toss potatoes and peppers with the oil and herb mixture.

Bake for 10 minutes or until potatoes are fork tender.

Sprinkle potatoes with parsley and Romano cheese.

Stir-Fried Orange Beef
4 Servings

1 tsp. cornstarch
1 cup orange juice
1 to 1 1/2 lbs. trimmed beef, sliced thin
1 to 2 T. of extra virgin olive oil
1 clove minced garlic
1 Tbsp grated fresh gingerroot
1/4 cup green onion, thinly sliced
1/4 cup bell pepper, thinly sliced

In small bowl, combine cornstarch and orange juice. Set aside. In wok, add beef, and olive oil. Stir-fry over high heat until beef is browned. Remove beef with slotted spoon. Set aside. Add garlic, gingerroot, onion, and bell pepper to oil remaining in the wok. Stir-fry 2 minutes. Add cornstarch/orange juice mixture. Simmer until thickened. Add beef and toss with sauce.

Can be served over noodles or rice.

Beef Brisket Stew
6 - 8 Servings

1 Beef Brisket (approx 3 lbs) trim fat
1 Tbsp extra virgin olive oil
3 lbs onions thinly sliced
2 Tbsp brown sugar
2 Tbsp minced garlic
1 Tbsp Tomato paste
½ cup dry red wine
1 cup Kitchen Basics Beef Broth
1 cup Kitchen Basics Chicken Broth
2 bay leaves
2 tsp thyme
1 Tbsp cider vinegar
6-8 red potatoes peeled and cut in quarters
1 15oz can of peas
6 carrots cut-up

Preheat oven to 300 degrees – move rack to the middle to accommodate an ovenproof Dutch oven pot.

Heat oil in pot over high heat. Sprinkle both sides of beef with salt. Cook brisket about 5 minutes until dark brown, turn over and brown other side for 5 minutes. Transfer brisket to a plate, set aside.

Reduce heat to medium, add onions, brown sugar and ¼ tsp salt. Stir frequently until softened and lightly browned, about 10 minutes. Stir in garlic and tomato paste for about a minute. Stir in beef broth, chicken broth, bay leaves and thyme. Add Brisket nestling in the liquid. Add potatoes and carrots in the last 1-1/2 hours.

Cover pot and place in oven. Cook until fork slides easily in and out of brisket, approximately 2-1/2 – 3 hours.

Add peas (you can add corn too) the last 15 minutes to heat up. Remove bay leaves before serving.

Banana Nut Bread

½ cup (1 stick) unsalted Land O' Lakes Butter
1 cup sugar
2 Large Eggs
3 ripe Bananas Mashed
2 Tbsp sour cream
1 tsp Arm & Hammer baking soda
2 cups unbleached all-purpose flour
1cup walnuts chopped

Set butter out at room temperature until softened.

Set eggs out at room temperature.

Preheat oven at 325 degrees

In a food processor or electric mixer, cream butter and sugar until creamy.

Add remaining ingredients to mixer. Place in a lightly greased (with butter) loaf pan and bake for 45 minutes to an hour, depending on your oven.

* I use 2 small loaf pans – freeze one – cut down my on baking.

Carrot Cake

2-1/2 cups unbleached all-purpose flour
1-1/4 tsp baking powder
1 tsp baking soda
1-1/4 tsp ground cinnamon
½ tsp nutmeg
1/8 tsp ground cloves
A pinch of ground allspice
½ tsp salt
1 pound of carrots shredded (I use my juicer to make carrot juice and use the pulp instead of peeling and shredding the carrots – about 3 cups).
1-1/2 cups sugar
½ cup packed light brown sugar
2 large eggs
1-1/2 cups safflower oil

Preheat oven at 350 degrees. Lightly grease (with butter) 13" x 9" baking pan lining the bottom of the pan with parchment paper also greased (this helps to remove from pan easily)

Whisk all the dry ingredients together and add shredded carrots in large mixing bowl. Set aside. In a food processor combine sugar and eggs and mix until frothy, and with machine running, slowly add the oil until all is combined. Remove from processor and pour into dry ingredients and carrots. Mix thoroughly. Pour into baking pan and bake for 35-40 minutes. Cool before removing from pan.

* I sometimes use 2 small loaf pans to cut slices instead of squares. I have one to freeze for another time. This cuts down on my baking.

Oatmeal & Raisin Cookies
Makes about 48 cookies

1¾ cups unbleached all-purpose flour
1 tsp baking soda
½ tsp salt
1 ¼ cups packed light brown sugar
2 sticks unsalted butter softened
½ cup granulated sugar
2 large eggs
2 Tbsp milk
2 tsp vanilla extract
2 ½ cups quick or old-fashioned oats
2 cups raisins
1 cup chopped walnuts (optional)

Preheat oven to 375 degrees. Line baking sheets with parchment paper.

Combine flour, baking soda and salt in small bowl and whisk together set aside.

Mix butter, and brown sugar in food processor or electric mixer until creamy. Add eggs one at a time, then add milk and vanilla extract. Scrape down bowl as necessary.

Gradually beat in flour and oats alternating mixture. Add raisins and then walnuts (optional).

Drop rounded Tbsp onto baking sheets. Bake for 9-10 minutes for chewy cookies or 12-13 minutes for crispy cookies. Place sheets on wire rack to cool.

Peanut Butter Cookies
Makes about 36 cookies

2 ½ cups unbleached flour
½ tsp baking soda
½ tsp baking powder
1 tsp salt
2 sticks unsalted butter softened
1 cup packed light brown sugar
1 cup crunchy peanut butter (no soybean or vegetable oil)
2 large eggs
2 tsp vanilla extract
1 cup dry-roasted peanuts chopped in food processor

Preheat oven to 350 degrees. Line baking sheets with parchment paper.

In a medium bowl, whisk together flour, baking soda, baking powder, and salt. Set aside.

In food processor or electric mixer, beat butter until creamy. Add the sugars, and beat until fluffy. Scrape bowl down as necessary.

Add peanut butter until completely mixed, then add eggs one at a time, then add vanilla extract.

Gently stir in flour a little at a time and when fully incorporated, add the peanuts stirring gently.

Make 2-inch balls flattened with fork in a crisscross design. Bake for 9-10 minutes until puffy and slightly browned on the outside, but not on top. They will look like they aren't done. Place on wire rack to cool.

Apple Crumb Pie

6 large Granny Smith apples peeled and cored and
sliced thin (6-7cups)
1/4 cup firmly packed light or dark brown sugar
½ cup raisins
1 Tbsp lemon juice
1 tsp ground cinnamon
3 Tbsp chopped walnuts (reserve some for topping)

For the Topping;

¼ cup (1/2 stick) butter cut into pieces
1/3 cup light or dark brown sugar

Preheat oven to 450 degrees

Prepare topping in a medium bowl, combine flour,
brown sugar. Place ingredients in a food processor or
blender, cut in butter until mixture resembles coarse
crumbs. Stir in reserved walnuts.

In a large bowl, combine brown sugar, apples, lemon
juice, raisins, walnuts, and cinnamon. Toss until well
coated. Spoon apples into pie pan.

Sprinkle with topping and bake for 20 minutes at 450
degrees, reduce oven temperature to 350 degrees for
about 40 minutes. Bake until bubbly. Place pie pan on
a wire rack to cool. Serve warm. Add a scoop of ice
cream!

Chocolate Pound Bundt Cake

3 cups all-purpose flour
½ cup unsweetened Dutch cocoa
1 tsp baking powder
¼ tsp salt
2 ¼ cups granulated sugar
¾ cup butter softened
3 large eggs
2 tsp vanilla extract
1 ¼ cups milk
1 cup chopped walnuts (optional)

Preheat oven to 325 degrees.

In a bowl combine flour, Dutch cocoa, baking powder, and salt. Whisk together, set aside.

In food processor or electric mixer beat sugar and butter at medium speed until well blended.

Add eggs blending completely one at a time, and then add vanilla extract.

Add flour mixture and milk alternated to sugar mixture. Mix in walnuts if desired.

Spoon batter into 12-cup Bundt pan greased with butter. Bake for 40 minutes or until toothpick inserted in cake comes out clean. Cool on wire rack for 10 minutes.

Chocolate Glaze for Bundt Cake

¾ cup powdered sugar
3 Tbsp unsweetened Dutch cocoa
2 Tbsp milk
½ tsp vanilla extract

Combine powdered sugar and 3 Tbsp Dutch cocoa.

Add 2 Tbsp milk and ½ tsp vanilla extract, whisk together and drizzle over cool cake.

- You can also just sprinkle powdered sugar on top of cake if you don't want a chocolate glaze.

CHAPTER 11

Allergy Info and Tips

I just thought I would add this section for adults and children who have other allergies.

Most importantly, I want to point out that exposure to chemical toxins in our foods today threatens the health and well being of mothers especially during the first twelve weeks of pregnancy and the affects these toxins play in their child's development.

It is estimated that 20% of Americans and especially children have allergies today. In the last twenty years there has been a 400% increases in allergies, 300% increase in asthma, with a 56% increase in asthma deaths, 400% increase in ADHD, and between 1,500 and 6,000% increase in autism!

The male/female ratio for food allergies is 2:1 and the male/female ratio for asthma is 3:1.

What are the symptoms of an allergic reaction?

When someone comes in contact with an allergen, the symptoms of a reaction may develop without warning, may be delayed, may happen as two episodes (biphasic) or may develop quickly then rapidly progress from mild to severe. The most dangerous symptoms include breathing difficulties and a drop in blood pressure or shock, which may result in loss of consciousness and even death. A person experiencing an allergic reaction may have **any** of the following symptoms:

- Trouble breathing, speaking or
- A drop in blood pressure, rapid heart beat, loss of consciousness
- Flushed face, hives or a rash, red and itchy skin

- Swelling of the eyes, face, lips, throat and tongue
- Anxiousness, distress, faintness, paleness, sense of doom, weakness
- Cramps, diarrhea, vomiting

Proteins in these eight major foods are estimated to cause 90 percent of the allergic reactions in the United States. ***The most common allergies are Milk, Eggs, Peanuts, Soy, Tree Nuts, Fish, Shellfish, and Wheat.***

Tips for Managing a Milk Allergy

Baking

Fortunately, milk is one of the easiest ingredients to substitute in baking and cooking. It can be substituted, in equal amounts, with water or fruit juice. (For example, substitute 1-cup milk with 1-cup water.)

Some Hidden Sources of Milk

- Deli meat slicers are frequently used for both meat and cheese products.
- Some brands of canned tuna fish contain casein, a milk protein.
- Many non-dairy products contain casein (a milk derivative), listed on the ingredient labels.
- Some meats may contain casein as a binder. Check all labels carefully.
- Many restaurants put butter on steaks after they have been grilled to add extra flavor. The butter is not visible after it melts.

Commonly Asked Questions:

Is goat milk a safe alternative to cow milk?

Goat's milk protein is similar to cow's milk protein and therefore, may cause a reaction in milk-allergic individuals. It is not a safe alternative.

Can I rely on kosher symbols to determine if a product is milk-free?

 The Jewish community uses a system of product markings to indicate whether a food is kosher, or in accordance with Jewish dietary rules.

There are two kosher symbols that can be of help for those with a milk allergy: a "D," or the word "dairy," on a label next to "K" or "U" (usually found near the product name) indicates presence of milk protein, and a "DE" on a label indicates the product was produced on equipment shared with dairy.

If the product contains neither meat nor dairy products, it is "pareve" (*parev, parve*). Pareve-labeled products indicate that the products are considered milk-free according to religious specifications. *Be aware that under Jewish law, a food product may be considered pareve even if it contains a very small amount of milk.* Therefore, a product labeled as pareve could potentially have enough milk protein in it to cause a reaction in a milk-allergic individual.

The following ingredients do **not** contain milk protein and need not be restricted by someone avoiding milk:

- Calcium lactate
- Lactic acid (however,

lactic acid starter culture may
contain milk)
- Calcium stearoyl lactylate
- oleoresin
- Cocoa butter
- Sodium lactate
- Cream of tartar
- Sodium stearoyl lactylate

Tips for Managing an Egg Allergy

Baking

For each egg, substitute one of the following in recipes. These substitutes work well when baking from scratch and substituting 1 to 3 eggs.

- 1 tsp. baking powder, 1 T. liquid, 1 T. vinegar
- 1 tsp. yeast dissolved in 1/4 cup warm water
- 1 1/2 T. water, 1 1/2 T. oil, 1 tsp. baking powder
- 1 packet gelatin, 2 T. warm water. Do not mix until ready to use.

Some Hidden Sources of Egg

- Eggs have been used to create the foam or milk topping on specialty coffee drinks and are used in some bar drinks.
- Some commercial brands of egg substitutes contain egg whites.
- Most commercially processed cooked pastas (including those used in prepared foods such as soup) contain egg or are processed on equipment shared with egg-containing pastas. Boxed, dry pastas are usually egg-free, but may be processed on equipment that is also used for

egg-containing products. Fresh pasta is sometimes egg-free, too. Read the label or ask about ingredients before eating pasta.

Some Hidden Sources of Peanuts

- Artificial nuts can be peanuts that have been deflavored and reflavored with a nut, such as pecan or walnut. Mandelonas are peanuts soaked in almond flavoring.
- Arachis oil is peanut oil.
- African, Chinese, Indonesian, Mexican, Thai, and Vietnamese dishes often contain peanuts or are contaminated with peanuts during the preparation process. Additionally, foods sold in bakeries and ice cream shops are often in contact with peanuts.
- Many brands of sunflower seeds are produced on equipment shared with peanuts.

Keep in Mind

- Studies show that most allergic individuals can safely eat peanut oil (not cold pressed, expelled, or extruded peanut oil - sometimes represented as gourmet oils). If you are allergic to peanuts, ask your doctor whether or not you should avoid peanut oil.
- Most experts recommend peanut-allergic patients avoid tree nuts as an extra precaution.
- Peanuts can be found in many foods and candies, especially chocolate candy. Check all labels carefully. Contact the manufacturer if you have questions.
- Peanuts can cause severe allergic reactions. If prescribed, carry epinephrine at all times. Here is more information about anaphylaxis:

Frequently Asked Questions

What is anaphylaxis?

Anaphylaxis is a sudden, severe, potentially fatal, systemic allergic reaction that can involve various areas of the body (such as the skin, respiratory tract, gastrointestinal tract, and cardiovascular system). Symptoms occur within minutes to two hours after contact with the allergy-causing substance but in rare instances, may occur up to four hours later. Anaphylactic reactions can be mild to life threatening. The annual incidence of anaphylactic reactions is about 30 per 100,000 persons, and individuals with asthma, eczema, or hay fever are at greater relative risk of experiencing anaphylaxis.

What are the common causes of anaphylaxis?

Common causes of anaphylaxis include:

- Food
- Medication
- Insect stings
- Latex

Less common causes include:

- Food-Dependent Exercise-Induced Anaphylaxis
- Idiopathic Anaphylaxis

Who is at risk for having an anaphylactic reaction?

Anyone with a previous history of anaphylactic reactions is at risk for another severe reaction. Individuals with food allergies (particularly allergies to shellfish, peanuts, and tree nuts) and asthma may be at increased risk for having a life-threatening anaphylactic reaction. A recent study showed that teens with food allergy and asthma appear to be at highest risk for a reaction because they are more likely to dine away from home, they are less likely to carry medications, and they may ignore or not recognize symptoms.

What are the symptoms of an anaphylactic reaction?

An anaphylactic reaction may begin with a tingling sensation, itching, or metallic taste in the mouth. Other symptoms can include hives, a sensation of warmth, asthma symptoms, swelling of the mouth and throat area, difficulty breathing, vomiting, diarrhea, cramping, a drop in blood pressure, and loss of consciousness. These symptoms may begin in as little as 5 to 15 minutes to up to 2 hours after exposure to the allergen, but life-threatening reactions may progress over hours.

Some individuals have a reaction, and the symptoms go away only to return two to three hours later. This is called a "biphasic reaction." Often the symptoms occur in the respiratory tract and take the individual by surprise.

How often does a person with peanut allergy also have a soy allergy?

Recent studies out of the University of London highlight the role that conventional soy (and soy formula) play in the development of the peanut allergy.

Because of these studies, the British Dietetic Association advises parents to avoid exposing infants under the age of one to soy. In France, parents are advised to avoid soy for children 0-3 years of age given the risk that it may present.[1]

The highest rate of allergy to soy was found in a study of 31 young children with peanut allergy, where 6.5 percent also had a soy allergy. Though soy and peanut are both beans (legumes), it is possible to be allergic to soy and not peanut, or to peanut and not soy. Why play Russian roulette?

How often do people with peanut allergies develop soy allergies, if they have been eating and tolerating soy?

According to studies, children between the ages of 10 and 19 are at a much higher risk of fatality due to allergies.

Many parents are unaware of the potential health risks that soy may present to children with peanut allergies.

Consider this – there was a segment on the Today Show October 25, 2007, about food allergies called "Edible Enemies."

This was about a thirteen-year-old girl named Emily who died after consuming a Sweet Onion Chicken-Teriyaki Wrap.

When Emily was two, she developed a peanut allergy after her father gave her a peanut butter cracker. She developed hives immediately, and her father gave her Benadryl and the symptoms subsided. So, here is a girl with only a known peanut allergy.

As she got older, when she came into contact with food that was exposed to nuts, she would have a tingling sensation on the back of her tongue. She immediately spit the food out, and threw up to get rid of whatever the allergen was. (I have done this too when I became nauseous, and wasn't sure all the ingredients were properly listed on the label).

Eventually, she developed swelling and asthma attacks in addition to the hives because of coming into contact with nuts.

Emily was very aware of her allergy. When she was in school, she was very cautious when it came to snacks. If her friends weren't sure whether the snack contained nuts, she tested it by putting her tongue on it. If she didn't have a reaction, she knew it was safe.
She did not carry an EpiPen. As far as they knew, she would have asthma attacks, and she carried an inhaler.

On April 13, 2007, Emily, her sister Elena, and her mother went shopping for a graduation dress. They stopped to have lunch in the food court at the mall. They chose a place that they had eaten at before because the only two items that had peanuts in them were cookies, and the rest of the menu was safe. Emily ordered the Sweet Onion Chicken-Teriyaki Wrap that she had eaten there so many times before without any problems. This of course is made with soy sauce.

They continued shopping. At first, while they were in a T-Shirt shop, Emily fell. They thought nothing of it. But, when they got to the store where Emily was going to have her ears pierced, Emily mentioned that she thought she messed her underwear when she fell, and wanted to check. When she returned 5 minutes later, she took two puffs of her inhaler and said she felt hot, and asked if her face looked red. Her mother reassured her that it wasn't and that they should leave.

Her new graduation dress that she was already wearing started to feel tight on her and she wanted to go change. So, the mother and Elena continued shopping. That's when the trouble started...a girl in the bathroom called the mother's cell phone and told her that Emily was having difficulty breathing. The immediately rushed to the bathroom and had her use the inhaler. CPR was performed immediately while Elena called 911. Emily became disoriented and wandered into the hallway. When her mother had her lay down, she passed out. At this time, she turned blue, and the mother heard a strange sound come out of her mouth.

The ambulance took Emily to the hospital, and 10 minutes later when the mother and sister arrived, the doctors told her they could not get her heart to start, and that they had given her all the medication they could to jumpstart her heart with no success.

Unfortunately, Emily was dead. But, to this day, the mother believes Emily died in the bathroom because of the last breath she heard her daughter take.

Is it worth having my peanut-allergic child who tolerates soy tested for soy?

Since both of these foods are beans, it is very common for a child with peanut allergy to test positive to soy, even though soy is tolerated with no symptoms in the beginning.

According to Dr. Yman, PhD of the Swedish National

Food Administraton, "Some sensitive children have "hidden" soy allergies that manifest for the first time with a severe – even fatal – reaction to even the low levels of "hidden" soy commonly found in processed food products. Those at the highest risk suffer from asthma as well as peanut allergy".[2]

This was just established in the story about Emily.

Until recently, I was able to tolerate peanuts, but this year I noticed that I was getting nauseous when I ate them. I took peanuts out of my diet and only eat walnuts now, although I can tolerate natural peanut butter. Even though my soy allergy developed later in life, I would rather play it safe and not eat soy even if I weren't allergic. If you have come this far in the book, you already know why soy should be avoided.

What is known about fatal reactions to soy in the context of peanut allergy?

In 1999, a study reported in a publication from Sweden identified four fatalities to foods that contained soy. The four individuals had peanut allergy and asthma, but had previously tolerated soy. The four deaths in Sweden were caused by hamburger (three cases) and kebob (one case). Though there was one fatality to soy reported in 1991, recent reports of 48 fatalities from the U.K. and 63 from the U.S. did not find a single fatality that was attributed to soy.

How do they really know that it wasn't attributed to soy? They don't! Remember, the doctors told me I had food poisoning! If I died, they never would have attributed it to eating soy.

Should my child with peanut allergy, who has

tolerated soy, avoid soy?

If my child were allergic to peanuts, knowing what I know now, I would definitely eliminate soy.

Some Hidden Sources of Tree Nuts

- Artificial nuts can be peanuts that have been deflavored and reflavored with a nut, such as pecan or walnut. Mandelonas are peanuts soaked in almond flavoring.
- Mortadella may contain pistachios.
- Tree nuts have been used in many foods, including barbecue sauce, cereals, crackers, and ice cream.
- Kick sacks, or hacky sacks, beanbags, and draft dodgers are sometimes filled with crushed nutshells.

Tips for Managing a Fish and/or Shellfish Allergy

Allergic reactions to fish and shellfish are commonly reported in both adults and children. It is generally recommended that individuals, who have had an allergic reaction to one species of fish, or positive skin tests to fish, avoid all fish. The same rule applies to shellfish. If you have a fish allergy but would like to have fish in your diet, speak with your allergist about the possibility of being tested with various types of fish.

Some Hidden Sources of Fish

- Caponata, a traditional sweet-and-sour Sicilian relish, can contain anchovies.
- Caesar salad dressings and steak or Worcestershire sauce often contain anchovies.

- Surimi (imitation crabmeat) contains fish.

Tips for Managing a Soy Allergy

Soybeans have become a major part of processed food products in the United States. Avoiding products made with soybeans is difficult (I know!), but not impossible.

Eliminate ALL processed and packaged foods, check frozen food labels (they all contain soybean oil), and forget about fast foods. When you eat in restaurants, make sure you ask what type of oil they use and if they use cooking spray for the grill – you'll have to forget about that too! You may not be able to eat their bread unless it's baked on the premises from scratch with butter (most restaurants have the bread shipped frozen-therefore saying it's baked fresh from the oven).

If I'm not sure, I order a salad without croutons, use olive oil & balsamic vinegar for dressing, or I bring my own salad dressing that I can trust.

As you have read, I have included a variety of recipes that I believe are nutritious. I enjoy meat, but there are still many benefits by just eliminating soy even if you don't eat meat.

Keep in Mind

- Soybeans and soy products are found in baked goods, canned tuna, cereals, crackers, infant formulas, sauces, and soups.
- At some brands of peanut butter lists soybean oil on the label (Sure, replace peanut oil with a cheap filler while you are paying for the expensive oil!)

Tips for Managing a Wheat Allergy

Baking

When baking with wheat-free flours, a combination of flours usually works best. Experiment with different blends to find one that will give you the texture you are trying to achieve.

Try substituting 1-cup wheat flour with one of the following:

- 7/8 cup rice flour
- 1-1/4 potato starch flour
- 2 cups corn flour

Keep in Mind

- Read labels carefully. At least one brand of hot dogs and one brand of ice cream contains wheat. It is listed on the label.
- Many country-style wreaths are decorated with wheat products.
- Some types of imitation crabmeat contain wheat.
- Wheat flour is sometimes flavored and shaped to look like beef, pork, and shrimp, especially in Asian dishes.[3]

[1, 2] http://www.allergykids.com
[3] http://www.foodallergy.org

CHAPTER 12

More Testimonials
Courtesy Of

www.soyonlineservice.co.nz

"I have been ill for several years and through research determined the cause to be soy, because in the past week I have been experiencing anaphylactic symptoms. My lips and cheeks have been swelling and my intestinal tract is in constant distress. I have had bouts of headaches, shortness of breath and lightheadedness. I have to lie down until it passes. Each time it appears to be worse than the last. I have found more information on various websites like yours to confirm my suspicions. I am shocked by the whole idea that there is next to nothing that I can eat. It is beyond my comprehension, why the government allows this!

"I was fed on soy formulas as an infant, and I have been a vegetarian for 40 years. For 30 years, I have had soy products as a source of protein, thinking that I was doing the right thing. Now I have severe hypothyroidism, and the clinical picture is not yet complete. I have more tests to take. I have battled a weight problem for ten years, and I now know why. I am angry about this soy deception!"

"Thank you! There are really people out there, who care about all this. The good news is my wife has been off the soy for 4 months now, and her goiter is gone. She feels much better and has more energy, and is more emotionally stable. . My tinnitus was also accompanied by a sudden allergy to wheat, corn, and soy - in fact just eating can now activate it. I was told to use flax oil to suppress an allergic reaction. Now I am stopping using I have found flax oil can have some of the same effects as soy. I hope my message also will validate somebody else with the same problem."

"I began drinking soy powder last year and just this week I have been diagnosed with Graves Disease. My daughter has Grave's Disease which I believe was caused by being fed soy milk in infancy."

"I have always been a relatively healthy woman. Now at 48 years old, I've been taking "Revival" products for about 3 years and recently began eating soy nuts. Although my TSH levels were normal, my sonogram found multiple goiters that I need to see an endocrinologist about. After reading many testimonials about soy effects, I've decided to completely stop consuming products with soy. I hope I will not need surgery."

"I have been researching the negative effects of soy for several reasons, For the past week, I have been on a soy based diet and have found that I gained 9 lbs in 7 days. This is highly unusual for my body. I went online to research if the change in my diet could be the cause and found the information about the ability of soy to depress the thyroid gland. I have removed soy from my diet, and I am hoping to reverse this sudden weight gain. More importantly, my vegan daughter gave birth to a son who was born with hypospadias (abnormality in which the opening of the urethra is on the underside, rather than at the end, of the penis), she researched the cause and only found information saying that the pesticides in her vegan diet may have been the cause. We now now have reason to believe it was her daily consumption of soy products. Her baby was scheduled to be weaned this week from breast milk & be put on soy formula, of course now that will not be the case. My son, who was allergic to milk when he was born 29 years ago, was put on prescription soy formula and is going for surgery to have his enlarged breasts reduced. Back then, my doctor never told me it was not tested, and my daughter's pediatrician just told her last week that soy formula was okay for our grandson. I am so surprised this soy issue is not in the forefront of the news and tests need to be done!"

"I was fed on soy formulas as an infant, and I have been a vegetarian for 40 years. For 30 years, I have had soy products as a source of protein, thinking that I was doing *the right thing. Now I have severe hypothyroidism, and the clinical picture is not yet complete. I have more tests to take. I have battled a weight problem for ten years, and I now know why. I am angry about this soy deception!"*

"I thought I was very healthy, and I live a healthy lifestyle (I never smoked, no alcohol, exercise frequently, low stress.) I'm 35 and have been a vegetarian for 25 years. I always eaten lots of soy, and increased my intake significantly the last 2 years because of increased physical activity (to ensure I received adequate protein). 5 years ago, my doctor noticed my thyroid was enlarged, but functioning normally. Now it's grown larger and I was diagnosed with papillary thyroid cancer. My preliminary research leads me to believe that soy was the cause of the thyroid enlargement and the subsequent cancer."

"My Grandparents were Seventh Day Adventists / Vegetarians. My grandfather was employed at Loma Linda Foods factory for most of his adult life with primarily processed soy based vegetarian foods, i.e., Veggie burgers. Not only do I have a thyroid problem (diagnosed at 17... I'm now 52) all of my cousins have thyroid problems as well."

"I am a 31 year old female and have always been healthy and fit. Last year, I thought I needed more protein (I suppose hearing all of the Atkins hype) and since I am not much of a meat eater, I started eating soy protein bars, such as Luna, and 'meatless' burgers. After only two weeks, I fell ill. I was completely exhausted, mentally foggy, and felt like I couldn't breathe. Just walking up the stairs made my heart race. I went to the doctor, and my blood work showed hypothyroid. The doctor asked me to come back for another test to determine the dosage of the thyroid medication that he intended to put me on. I found several articles telling of the dangers of soy and the effects it can have on the thyroid. I tossed out all of the

soy stuff and within a few days, I felt 100% better. And when I went back several days later for the second blood test, guess what? Thyroid function was completely normal. I truly believe that the soy products are what caused the problem. I no longer eat soy products and I've been fine."

"I have been dieting with Jenny Craig for the past 3 months. I also am being treated for depression & hypothyroidism. Recently, due to "funny feelings" I investigated the soy content of this food & found that most of their foods have some too much soy. I have been satisfied with my weight loss (17 lbs thus far) and the ease with which the food is available and planned, but I am uncertain about the effect the quantities in these foods may be having on my "ailments." I don't know if soy is the main culprit or I may be contributing to my problems by ingesting soy products in Jenny Craig meals."

"I wasn't fed soy infant formula, however I have been a huge consumer of soymilk & soy protein powder over the last 20+ years. I am a vegetarian and I am 45 years old. I have suffered with hypothyroidism for the last 2 years. I am a physician and I have noticed in my practice an increasing incidence of thyroid disease, primarily in my female patients."

"I am very grateful for the information you have provided and I think someone should get on the bandwagon and tell people about the dangers of Soy products. We knew smoking was dangerous, but we never knew the addictive properties of the cigarettes. Now we know after 30 years of arguing about it and the cigarette industry is being held accountable for their deceptions. Maybe if the Soy industry is threatened with the same legal ramifications they will try to better educate the public of the dangers of soy and thyroid patients."

"Thank you so much for your article that connects soy products to Thyroid, especially soymilk with Isoflavone powder. I am suffering from Hypothyroid for many years, and am taking medication to balance the hormone function. Recently I read an online promotional article for the Isoflavone product and the benefits women at Menopause can gain from taking it. I bought this product 3 months ago and started to take it daily. I took a blood test a few days ago to determine the level of my TCH. My physician called me today and told me to come immediately to his clinic since the level of my TCH increased dramatically- from 5 to 11."

"I am 32 years old and was diagnosed with hypothyroidism three weeks ago. I began consuming soy in earnest about four years ago in response to consumer information claiming that soy may help to decrease one's chances of developing breast cancer, heart disease and more. My mother died of breast cancer when she was 39 years old and I have been diligent in eating an extremely healthy diet geared towards maintaining optimal health and disease prevention. During the past four years, I incorporated numerous food products in my diet that were primarily soy based. Also, I regularly consumed a large amount of soy protein powder that I added to shakes and food during cooking and baking. The past four years I consumed at least 40 - 60 mgs of soy a day. I now have a goiter, and hypothyroidism and severe anemia. Based on the information I have read about soy subsequent to this diagnosis, I have a great concern that the soy may indeed have played a large part in generating this thyroid disorder, if not be the direct cause."

"I was just diagnosed with Graves Disease today. In 1997, 6 months after starting Tamoxifen, I was becoming confused often. I thought this was because I was in menopause and needed more hormones. I started with two servings of soy per day, and then I have increased my

soy protein consumption to 3 or 4 servings a day. It does appear that the soy caused my hyperthyroidism."

"My story is just like everyone else's. My "former" doctor attributed everything to old age.... (I don't consider age 53 old.) I switched to an alternative doctor and the first thing he told me was he does not recommend soy products. In the past two years, I went from an energetic, happy-go-lucky, healthy person. I figured that I needed more protein, and meat wasn't good for you, so I switched to soy: soy protein shakes, tofutti ice cream, soy milk, Luna bars (and others), soy cereal, cookies, you name it - if it was soy, I ate it. I began to get run down...had severe leg cramps, muscle twitching, tinnitis, joint aches and stiffness, gastrointestinal problems, and worst of all, hair loss. I got colds and bronchitis one after another. I couldn't concentrate long enough to exercise. I am now on thyroid (naturally made) pills, and have been off soy for two weeks. My muscles and joints don't hurt, I'm getting my "groove" back, and I am exercising. My bronchitis is gone, and so are my tinnitus, eyelid twitching, and leg cramps. This seems to be an epidemic, and the public is greatly fooled by people touting the advantages of consuming soy. I am going back to eating real, whole, natural foods as our elders ate. My "miracle" food, turned into a nutritional nightmare."

"I am a monk and completed a long retreat that was terminated early due to health problems. I went to the doctor and was told that my thyroid was not functioning at all!" I never had thyroid problems and was a bit shocked. I heard of women experiencing this problem. I researched the Internet and discovered the connection with soy products. At the retreat, my staple was tempeh and tofu supplemented by bread that I baked with lots of soy flour. I did not know that this could be a problem"

"While being on a nutrition/exercise program, it was

recommended that I increase my intake of protein, so I thought, what better way to do so, than take a Soy protein shake each day? I started taking Soy protein shakes, with added isoflavones, at least 4 times a day in order to meet my daily protein requirements. After 14 weeks I began to symptoms of increased heart rate/heart palpitations, diminished mental capacity, nausea, gastro intestinal upset/problems, prolonged menstrual bleeding, headaches, dizziness/vertigo, increasing tiredness, and lack of energy usually within 20 minutes of consuming a shake each time. I have concluded after much research that soy has to be the center of my problems. I will no longer use Soy or Soy based products in any capacity."

"I am a fairly healthy 36 year old female, run about 20 miles a week, and walk about 5 miles a week and do light toning & cardio exercises. I fell in love with these "Zone" bars, which contain 16 grams of soy protein per bar, approx. 32 mg. of soy isoflavones. I began eating these bars as meal replacements, but have gotten down to eating only 1 or 2 bars daily. I was diagnosed with hypothyroid. Since I went on the Synthroid, I can barely run over a mile without experiencing dizziness & nausea. I was contributing all of my problems to the Synthroid and researched it on the Internet and learned it's probably the soy that has caused my problems in the first place! I have had considerable hair thinning, trouble maintaining, and losing weight, despite my "healthy" diet & exercise regimen. I am tired all the time and experience feelings of depression more than not. Today I quit both my Synthroid as well as the Zone bars - I don't feel any different yet, and don't expect to feel any different for quite some time.

"For two years I ingested large amounts of soy on a daily diet: soymilk, tofu, soy cheese, soy burgers and soy yogurt. Having milk sensitivity I naturally substituted soy as a source of protein. Last fall I had a medical crisis: my TSH soared to 25.50; lost more than half my hair;

developed large uterine fibroids; evidenced rapid cellular growth (benign) on both breasts; and lost elasticity in my muscles, including my bladder causing urinary incontinence. I am 43 years of age. Upon eliminating the soy, my TSH is now 1.4 (I had to be placed on a therapeutic regimen of 75 mcg of Synthroid) and my alopecia has reversed. I suffered needlessly and if not for my hair loss I would probably still be using soy. It was the alopecia that gave me great cause for alarm."

"I am a 30-year-old vegetarian who has been taking in around 40-50 grams of soy protein a day. I have recently started having problems with heart palpitations and weight gain. I am on the Weight Watchers points system and I have gained 11 lb. in 2 1/2 months. I have been very disturbed by this gain, knowing that I am exercising 5-6 days a week and staying very active every day. Everyone else on WW is losing except for me it seems. My grandmother was diagnosed with thyroid disease many years ago and I seem to have all the symptoms such as, weight gain, palpitations, memory loss. I read articles that made me aware that soy is to blame. I don't know if I have already damaged my thyroid, but I am going to stop my soy intake today!"

"I had thyroid problems as a child, and was treated with medication then. As an adult, I didn't require any medication for years. I began drinking lots of soymilk, eating tofu and enjoying miso, plus taking a vitamin, which contained soy. Lo' and behold, I started having thyroid problems again. I now take medication again. I have completely discontinued all soy products and any other phytoestrogen products. So far, I am still required to take medication, but hopefully, my thyroid will become balanced again. I am so very pleased to find your web site. I have been trying to explain to many women the dangers of using soy products as a miracle solution to everything without consideration of their age, conditions, etc."

"I would like to get the word out that folk who are already Hypothyroids should not consume soy because it blocks their medication from being effective. I have already proved that by coming off soy my TSH that I had extreme difficulty getting below 5+ is now down to 0.03! My doctor is so thrilled he is now telling all his thyroid patients to come off soy. As well as that, I am NOW finally losing weight after years of putting it on. My 31 year old daughter had developed a goiter around 10 years ago and now she is off soy and the goiter had all but disappeared."

"I am 45 years of age, female, have developed a goiter, and have tested positive for thyroiditis antibodies. The only thing that has changed in my diet over the past few years has been consumption of soy, which has been high because I have been taking Genisoy protein powder (with isoflavones) on a daily basis for all this time. I check photos of myself over this period, and noticed that the goiter appeared only after a few months of starting the protein powder. Unfortunately, I have also been eating cereal supplemented with soy, as well as tofu and soy sauce. My thyroid condition has come as a shock to me, and I am taking the issue up with my doctor, who recommended the diet in the first place. I will also be contacting a journalist with a view to writing an article for the mainstream press in order to help other women before it's too late for them."

"I am a 47 year old woman in peri-menopause. I was suffering with very intense hot flashes, and night sweats so I began searching for relief. After reading, going to my health food store, and speaking to several individuals I decided to try soy and a multi-herb supplement. In July 1999 I started taking two 40 mg capsules of Soyplus and six 400 mg capsules of Vitex 40 Plus daily. Almost immediately I began gaining weight. I researched the herbs in the supplement and found that black cohosh *causes weight gain. I kept taking the herbs. After I gained 25 pounds in five months I stopped taking the herbs (but still took the soy). I had a medical checkup and my blood work showed hypothyroidism."*

"I am a 49 year old woman. About a year ago, my GYN tested my hormone levels and informed me I was menopausal. He put me on estriadol/progesterone. Not liking the way I felt or the perceived risk of hormones, I stopped taking them. I decided after reading all of the hype about soy to try it. Please understand, I never had a weight problem, sleep problem, thinning hair, mood disorder before this. I began taking a soy tablet of 50 mg per day. Although I worked out everyday and ate a healthy diet, I started battling with my weight. 7 months later, I gained approximately 10 pounds; my hair was falling out, and was having terrible bouts with mood swings and temper. I was convinced I needed to stay on the soy. So convinced, I bought the Revival Soy package. I took it for a couple of weeks, everyday and convinced myself I felt better and was losing weight, when in fact, facial hair was appearing, my hot flashes had returned and I was gaining weight. I stopped. I had major surgery in February and had 10 weeks of at home recuperation. During the first four weeks, I didn't take any vitamins, supplements, or soy. All of a sudden, I had lost 8 lbs. BUT thinking I need to "get my body healthy," I began the Revival Soy again. I stayed on it for one month. During that time, my mood swings were horrible, my hair started falling out, and hot flashes were back and gained back the weight. So, I stopped the Revival again. But this time, nothing happened. After reading your website, it is apparent to me that NOTHING will happen because my expensive vitamins have soy in them. They are going in the trash tonight! I only hope and pray my thyroid is not destroyed."

"I am 21 years old, and about 12 months ago I developed a lump in my right breast, I had the lump checked out and it was confirmed as nothing but fibro glandular swelling, however it was quite painful, I was also suffering fatigue, weight gain and poor libido. The doctor recommended I start HRT. I was nervous about taking a drug for menopausal women. My Pharmacist suggested that I take phytoestrogen/ isoflavones through natural menopausal supplements and soy consumption. I was already using soy to reduce my daily dairy intake. I was happy to start these natural supplements hoping that my painful breast lump would go down. The lump however got larger and more painful. I guess I did not connect that with the soy because I was told it would reduce these symptoms so I took even more soy. I drank up to a liter of soy milk, ate a tub of soy yogurt per day, had miso soup every other day, linseed bread, and ate soy cereal. My lump got even larger (about the size of a golf ball), and the pain so unbearable I couldn't wear certain lingerie. I was diagnosed as fibrocystic breast disease. I was connected to a hormone website and I was told to stop taking the contraceptive pill (which I have been taking for approx 5 years) and to reduce/stop the soy intake as I was suffering from an estrogen excess. And what relief! I stopped taking the pill only 5 days ago, ceased my soy intake about 2 weeks ago, and for at least the past week the lump has considerably reduced in size and the pain has almost stopped- which suggests that it may be connected with my soy intake, because the symptoms began to clear before I stopped taking the pill. I believe this could be due to my soy intake.

Campaign For Healthy Living

If you want to make a difference, contact the companies below and let them know that you will not be fooled with unhealthy "no trans fats" and cheap fillers for their higher profits anymore! They are all switching to soybean oil, and that is not a healthy alternative. Now is your chance to speak out. Don't you want your families and generations to come to live a long and healthy life? Please help me spread the word.
Thank you.

Fast Food Companies

McDonald's Corporation
1 KrocDrive
OakBrook, IL 60521
(708) 575-3000, (708) 575-5512 fax

Burger King Corporation
PO Box52078
Miami, FL 33142
(305) 378-7011, (305) 378-7262 fax

Pizza Hut Worldwide
9111 East Douglas
Wichita, KS 67207
(619) 681-9000, (619) 681-9869 fax

Taco Bell Worldwide
17901 Von Karmon
Irvine, CA 92714
(714) 863-4500

Wendy's
PO Box 256
Dublin, OH 43017
(614) 764-3100, (614) 764-3459 fax

Hardee's
1233 Hardee's Blvd.
Rocky Mount, NC 27804
(919) 977-2000, (919) 977-8655 fax

Kentucky Fried Chicken
PO Box 32070
Louisville, KY 40232
(502) 456-8300

Little Caesar Enterprise, Inc.
2211 Woodward Avenue
Detroit, MI 4820 1-3400
(313) 983-6000, (313) 983-6197 fax

International Dairy Queen, Inc.
PO Box 39286
Minneapolis, MN 55439-0286
(612) 830-0200, (612) 830-0480 fax

Food Processing Companies

Nestlé USA, Inc.
800 N. Brand Blvd.
Glendale CA 91203
(818) 549-6000, (819) 549-6952 fax
(Carnation, Raisinettes, Butterfinger,
Chunky, Stouffers and Lean Cuisine)

Philip Morris
120 Park Avenue
New York, NY 10017
(212) 880-5000
(Kraft, General Foods, Entenmanns,
Stove Top Stuffing, and Cool Whip)

Grand Metropolitan
30 St. James Square
London, England SW1Y4RR
(44-71) 321-6000
(Pillsbury and Hungry Jack)

RJR Nabisco
1301 Ave. of the Americas
New York, NY 10019
(212) 258-5600
(Nabisco, Fleishmann's, Planter's Peanuts,
Stella d'Oro and Chun King)

Sara Lee
Three First National Plaza
Chicago, IL 60602
(312) 726-2600
(Baked goods)

Frito-Lay
7701 Legacy Drive
Dallas, TX75035
(214) 351-7000
(Chips and snack foods)

CPC International
International Plaza Box 8000
Englewood Cliffs, NJ 07632
(201) 894-4000, (201) 894-2186 fax
(Bran' nola, Arnold's, Hellman's, Mazola
and Skippy)

Kellogg's
PO Box 3 599
Battle Creek, Michigan 49016
(619) 961-2000
(Eggo, Le Gout and Mrs. Smith's)

Campbell Soup
Campbell Place
Camden, NJ 08103
(609) 342-4800
(Swanson & Pepperidge Farm)

Continental Baking Company
Checkerboard Square
St. Louis, MO 63164
(314) 392-4700

UTZ Quality Foods
900 High Street
Hanover, PA 17331
(717) 637-6644

Quaker Oats Company
321 North Clark Street
Chicago, IL 60610
(312) 222-7111
(Quaker Oats & Aunt Jemima)

Proctor and Gamble
PO Box 599
Cincinnati, OH 45201
(513) 983-1100

VanDen Bergh Foods Company
2200 Cabot Drive
Lisle, IL 60532
(800) 955-5532
(Imperial Margarine, I Can't Believe
It's Not Butter, Ragu & BakerSource)

Lance
PO Box 32368
Charlotte, NC 28232
(704) 554-1421
(Cookies & Crackers)

Keebler Company
One Hollow Tree Lane
Elmhurst, IL 60126
(708) 782-2630
(Cookies & Crackers)

Sunshine Biscuits, Inc.
100 Woodbridge Center Drive
Woodbridge, NJ 07095
(908) 855-4000
(Cookies & Crackers)

Printed in the United Kingdom by
Lightning Source UK Ltd., Milton Keynes
142428UK00001B/207/P